Diarrhoea
and **constipation**
in **geriatric practice**

This textbook provides a practical and comprehensive account of the management of diarrhoea and constipation in the elderly. These common disorders in the elderly are not only a burden in themselves but are often manifestations of a more serious underlying illness: thus, effective diagnosis and treatment are essential to improve quality of life.

Many important conditions are associated with diarrhoea. The text includes updates on pathogenesis, diagnosis and treatment, and highlights the vulnerability of the elderly with regard to acquiring diarrhoea and its complications.

The aetiology of diarrhoea is explained, including infections of the gastrointestinal tract, and systemic diseases of which diarrhoea is a manifestation. Diverse disciplines are spanned: from immunology and physiology to microbiology, nutrition and psychiatry.

The aetiology, diagnosis and treatment of constipation ʒ dealt with, emphasizing practical management issues.

The book is aimed at geriatricians, general practitiᴄ   allied health workers.

Diarrhoea
and **constipation**
in **geriatric practice**

Edited by

Ranjit N. Ratnaike

MD, FRACP, FAFPHM

Department of Medicine, The University of Adelaide,
The Queen Elizabeth Hospital,
Woodville, South Australia

Foreword by

Gary R. Andrews

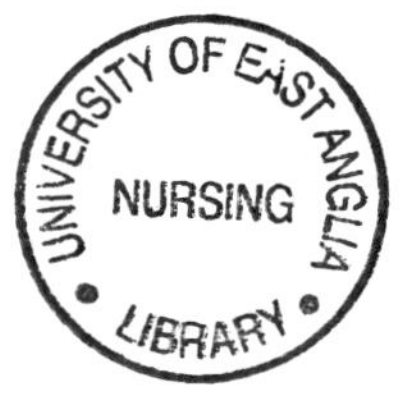

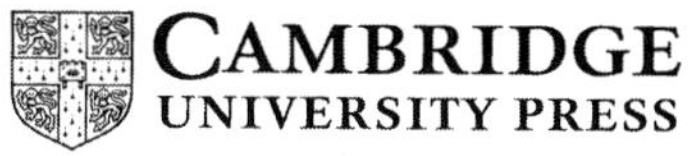

CAMBRIDGE
UNIVERSITY PRESS

PUBLISHED BY THE PRESS SYNDICATE OF THE UNIVERSITY OF CAMBRIDGE
The Pitt Building, Trumpington Street, Cambridge, United Kingdom

CAMBRIDGE UNIVERSITY PRESS
The Edinburgh Building, Cambridge CB2 2RU, UK   www.cup.cam.ac.uk
40 West 20th Street, New York, NY 10011–4211, USA   www.cup.org
10 Stamford Road, Oakleigh, Melbourne 3166, Australia
Ruiz de Alarcón 13, 28014 Madrid, Spain

First published 1999

Printed in the United Kingdom at the University Press, Cambridge

Typeset in Adobe Minion 10.5/14 pt. in QuarkXPress™ [SE]

A catalogue record for this book is available from the British Library

Library of Congress Cataloguing in Publication data
Diarrhoea and constipation in geriatric practice/
edited by Ranjit N. Ratnaike.
     p.   cm.
Includes index.
ISBN 0 521 65388 6 (pbk.)
1. Diarrhea in old age.   2. Constipation in old age.
I. Ratnaike, Ranjit N.
[DNLM: 1. Diarrhea – therapy.   2. Diarrhea – in old age.
3. Constipation – therapy.   4. Constipation – in old age.   WI 407
M2658 1999]
RC862.D5M365   1999
618.97′63427–dc21   98–46889 CIP
DNLM/DLC
for Library of Congress

ISBN 0 521 65388 6 paperback   # 1083133

Every effort has been made in preparing this book to provide accurate and up-to-date information which is
in accord with accepted standards and practice at the time of publication. Nevertheless, the authors, editors
and publisher can make no warranties that the information contained herein is totally free from error, not
least because clinical standards are constantly changing through research and regulation. The authors,
editors and publisher therefore disclaim all liability for direct or consequential damages resulting from the
use of material contained in this book. Readers are strongly advised to pay careful attention to information
provided by the manufacturer of any drugs or equipment that they plan to use.

For

Stephanie Kathlean

Contents

Contributors

Joseph E. Buttery
PhD
Department of Clinical Chemistry,
The Queen Elizabeth Hospital, Woodville,
South Australia,
Australia

James McA. Cooper
MB, BS, PhD
Modbury Hospital, Modbury,
South Australia,
Australia

Adrian G. Cummins
BSc (Med), MD, PhD, FRACP
Gastroenterology Unit,
The Queen Elizabeth Hospital, Woodville,
South Australia,
Australia

Ian Darnton-Hill
MB, BS, Dip Nutri Diet MPH, MSc (Med),
    FAFPHM
Regional Office for the Western Pacific,
World Health Organization,
United Nations Avenue,
1099 Manila,
Philippines

R. Logan Faust
MD
Division of Gastroenterology,
University of California, Davis Medical.
    Center,
Sacramento, California,
USA

William M.H. Goh
MB, BS, FRANZCP
Department of Psychiatry,
The University of Adelaide,
The Queen Elizabeth Hospital,
Woodville, South Australia,
Australia

Sally Hudson
B App Sc Adv Nur (N Ed), B Ng (Hons),
    RN, RM
Royal District Nursing Service of SA Inc.,
Glenside, South Australia,
Australia

Terry E. Jones
B Pharm, Dip Ed
Pharmacy Department,
The Queen Elizabeth Hospital, Woodville,
South Australia,
Australia

Tina Koch
RN, CHC, BA, PhD, FRCNA
School of Nursing,
The Flinders University,
Bedford Park, South Australia,
Australia

Peter J. Lawson
FAIMS, MASM
Department of Microbiology,
The Queen Elizabeth Hospital, Woodville,
South Australia,
Australia

David F.M. Looke
MB, BS, FRACP, FRCPA
Department of Infectious Diseases and
    Clinical Microbiology,
The Queen Elizabeth Hospital, Woodville,
South Australia,
Australia

Ludomyr J. Mykyta
MB, BS, MRCP, FRACP, FACRM
Rehabilitation Medicine,
Aged Care,
Western Domiciliary Care & Rehabilitation
    Service,
Woodville Park, South Australia,
Australia

N.V.K. Nair
MB, BS, MSc, MPH
Regional Office for the Western Pacific,
World Health Organization,
United Nations Avenue,
1099 Manila,
Philippines

Ranjit N. Ratnaike
MD, FRACP, FAFPHM
Department of Medicine,
The University of Adelaide,
The Queen Elizabeth Hospital, Woodville,
South Australia,
Australia

Ian Roberts-Thomson
MD, FRACP
Gastroenterology Unit,
The Queen Elizabeth Hospital, Woodville,
South Australia,
Australia

Pamela F. Sando
RN, CCRN, Dip App Sci, BN
Staff Development Education,
The Royal Adelaide Hospital,
North Terrace, Adelaide, South Australia,
Australia

Seppo K. Suomela
MD
Regional Office for the Western Pacific,
World Health Organization,
United Nations Avenue,
1099 Manila,
Philippines

David J. Torpy
MB, BS, PhD, FRACP
Endocrinology Unit,
The Queen Elizabeth Hospital, Woodville,
South Australia,
Australia

Anil B. Utturkar
MD, DMRE, FRACR
Department of Radiology,
The Queen Elizabeth Hospital, Woodville,
South Australia,
Australia

Michael C. Woodward
MB, BS, FRACP
Aged Care Services,
Heidelberg Repatriation Hospital,
Heidelberg West, Victoria,
Australia

Preface

Diarrhoea and Constipation in Geriatric Practice is a text primarily for geriatricians and other health professionals, such as general practitioners, who are involved in the care of the elderly. The elderly comprise a significant and increasing segment of the population in both the industrialized and the developing countries. The problem of diarrhoea and constipation in this aging population is likely to attract increasing attention. The extent of these problems and their social and physical implications are perhaps not sufficiently recognized. The common problem of constipation in the elderly is discussed, with emphasis on practical management issues.

The text covers the important conditions associated with diarrhoea and updates the information on pathogenesis, diagnosis and treatment. The vulnerability of the elderly with regard to acquiring diarrhoea and to the complications is also highlighted.

There is a greater emphasis on diarrhoea in the text. This is because the aetiology is extensive, encompassing many infections of the gastrointestinal tract (which are relevant in the developing world) and includes systemic diseases of which diarrhoea is a manifestation. Diverse disciplines are spanned: from immunology and physiology to microbiology, nutrition and psychiatry.

The separate chapter on coeliac disease is to highlight the importance of this condition. The diagnosis may sometimes not be considered in the elderly.

The aim of this book is to provide information to help understand the many facets of diarrhoea and to assist in the prevention, diagnosis and management of diarrhoea in the elderly.

Increasingly, the emphasis is on the care of the elderly person in the community rather than in an institution, and the role of the nurse practitioner is of great importance. Chapter 19 addresses a variety of issues which would be useful to nurses involved in the care of the elderly.

It is hoped that this text will provide comprehensive information to manage successfully the common problems of diarrhoea and constipation in the elderly with a view to improving quality of life.

Acknowledgments

Many of my colleagues may have felt their patience and friendship tested by my frequent requests for information and opinion on a variety of matters which have ranged from physiology to philology. I am indebted to the following who helped in a variety of ways: Dr Sylvia Barber, Dr Clive Beng, Mr Colin Hentschke, Mr Manohar Hullan, Ms Sue Millard, Dr John Norman, Mr Alan Oakes, Dr John Pierides, Ms Sue Dowsett and Ms Sue Rockliff. I would like to thank Ms Tracy Merlin for her help in a number of areas and Mr Austin Milton for checking the final manuscript.

I am most grateful to Mrs Mary Denys for her work in preparing the manuscript and I am indebted to her for her tolerance and unfailing cheerfulness despite such a heavy workload.

The contributors to this text were, without exception, a great pleasure to work with.

The spouses of editors and authors of books, from what I have read in 'Acknowledgments' in other texts, must belong to a group with the qualities of great patience, tolerance and a sense of humour. My wife, Stephanie, has exhibited all of these virtues and more. I thank her for drawing Figure 3.1, and I am particularly grateful to her and our children for their forbearance and encouragement. Finally, I am indebted to Peter Silver and to Roy Baker of Cambridge University Press for their assistance with this text.

Foreword

Older persons are of increasing importance in almost every arena of medical practice. In developed countries people aged 65 years and over constitute 12 to 18 per cent of the general population but account for around 30 to 40 per cent of the consumption of health care services. The global increase in total numbers of older persons is astonishing; by the year 2025 there will be more than 800 million people aged 65 years and over in the world, two thirds of them in developing countries.

The older person has a fundamental right to expect and receive high quality medical care including, where appropriate, the application of the most recent technological advances available.

There is a pressing need for more detailed texts that deal comprehensively, and in depth, with particular aspects of medicine in old age.

Medical practitioners in almost all situations encounter a growing proportion of older persons in daily practice, often presenting differently from the standard textbook description of disease and frequently with multiple and complex disorders. Improved information on disease in old age, and education and training in the practice of best medicine in providing care for the older person, is critical at every level.

This book, written by a group of highly skilled and informed practitioners, covers an important and sometimes neglected area of health in old age. Its publication during the 1999 International Year of Older Persons is remarkably timely. It reminds us of the need to deal not only with the rhetoric and broad pronouncements on the importance of individual and population aging, but also to focus on the most basic and practical issues associated with achieving good medical practice in old age. The topics covered in this book are relevant not only to specialist geriatricians but to all medical and health care providers who are involved with the care of older persons.

Gary R. Andrews
Director, Centre for Ageing Studies,
Flinders University of South Australia; and
Special Advisor on Ageing to the United Nations

Part I

Defences of the aging gastrointestinal tract

Nonimmune defences of the aging gut

Ranjit N. Ratnaike

In the elderly the nonimmunological defences of the gastrointestinal tract are an essential defence mechanism to protect the host against enteric infections. These defences, with aging, are compromised by a variety of external influences.

The nonimmunological defences are the first line of protection against enteric pathogens. The stomach, small intestine and colon are involved. Toxins are expelled by vomiting; pathogens are destroyed by gastric acid. The contact of toxins and bacteria with the small intestinal mucosa is minimized by the motility of the intestine. Pathogens which reach the colon are faced with a hostile population of commensal organisms, unwilling to relinquish their mutually beneficial relationship with their host.

Gastric defences

Vomiting

Vomiting ejects gastric contents and is the most primitive defence mechanism of the gastrointestinal tract. This powerful mechanism for 'clearing' and 'cleansing' gastric contents occurs through vigorous retrograde propulsion and is the most prominent feature of food poisoning due to ingested toxins.

The vomiting centre in the medulla is stimulated via afferent nerve impulses from chemoreceptors in the first part of the duodenum, which are sensitive to emetic substances. The ablation of this area eliminates vomiting despite the ingestion of these substances. Recent work points to an area separate from the vomiting centre in the medulla, called the area postrema or chemoreceptor trigger zone (CTZ), that is sensitive to substances circulating in the blood that cause vomiting.

Gastric acid

The gastric acid barrier is an important defence mechanism against enteric pathogens. Most organisms that cause diarrhoea are acquired orally and are susceptible to gastric acid. Rarely, infections occur due to anal intercourse, instrumentation and unsterile enemas for 'colonic irrigation'.

Gastric juice consists of water, hydrochloric acid, bicarbonate, inorganic ions (mainly sodium and potassium) and mucus, diluted with swallowed salivary juice. The pH of gastric acid and bacterial counts in the stomach show a close correlation. In normal subjects the gastric pH is usually below pH 4, a critical level for protection against enteric pathogens, and the stomach is virtually sterile. At pH 4–5 bacteria in the saliva are present in the stomach. A pH greater than 5 allows bacterial, viral and protozoan pathogens to survive.

The important relationship between gastric acidity and bacterial survival is demonstrated by experiments on human volunteers. A 10 000-fold increase in susceptibility to *Vibrio cholerae* occurs when 2 g of sodium bicarbonate is administered with the bacterial dose. The minimal infectious dose of 10^3–10^4 *Salmonella typhi* is significantly reduced by the simultaneous ingestion of sodium bicarbonate. The risk of diarrhoea due to enteric pathogens increases as the pH of gastric acid rises.

Decreased acid production may be part of the aging process and achlorhydria occurs in up to 20 per cent of subjects over the age of 60 years. A recent study challenges the view that decreased acid production is a primary feature of the aging process. Hurwitz et al. (1997) found in their elderly subjects that decreased acid secretion reflected atopic gastritis. Factors which decrease gastric acidity are pernicious anaemia, atrophic gastritis, malnutrition, gastric carcinoma and the WDHA syndrome (watery diarrhoea, hypokalaemia and achlorhydria). *Helicobacter pylori* infection may result in atrophic gastritis which could decrease the parietal cell mass to cause reduced acid output.

In the elderly the protective effect of the gastric acid barrier is further decreased by drugs used to decrease acid production or neutralize acid already secreted in the treatment of peptic ulceration, severe gastro-oesophageal reflux and the Zollinger–Ellison syndrome (H_2 receptor antagonists, proton pump inhibitors and antacids). The elevation of gastric pH with cimetidine correlates with increased numbers of gastric microflora, and ceasing treatment restores normal gastric pH and sterility within six hours. Diarrhoea has been associated with cimetidine therapy in 3 to 12 per cent of patients. Omeprazole therapy results in bacterial overgrowth in 53 per cent of patients. In the elderly, the use of H_2 blockers is reported to be a significant risk factor for carriage of *Clostridium difficile*.

Other drugs which decrease acid production are anticholinergic drugs and tricyclic antidepressant drugs.

Surgical procedures, such as gastrectomy and vagotomy to decrease gastric acidity before the era of effective oral therapy, are associated with diarrhoea. As soon as seven days after a surgical procedure for acid reduction, significant bacterial colonization occurs and persists up to six months. Gastric stasis and disordered small bowel motility are contributory. The association between partial gastrectomy and bacterial overgrowth of pathogens in the stomach and upper small intestine and diarrhoea is well documented (see Chapter 15).

Small intestinal defences

The small intestine is a complex multifunctional organ involved in host defence. It receives gastric juice, secretes enzymes, bile and pancreatic juice and is responsible for food digestion and absorption and for the movement of luminal contents to the colon. In addition, by the strategies discussed below the small intestine protects itself from agents that adversely affect its delicate lining, the mucosa, and ultimately the host.

Motility

Motility of the gastrointestinal tract is an important defence mechanism against enteric pathogens and substances harmful to the host.

The environment of the small intestine is continuously changing and presents a hostile milieu to pathogens. Enzymes and secretions to aid digestion that are harmful to pathogens are continuously produced; enterocytes on which bacteria may adhere are constantly shed and replaced; the mucus barrier is swept away and replenished. The motility of the small intestine assists in all these activities to protect the host.

There is no evidence of significantly altered small intestinal motility associated with the aging process. Intestinal motility is associated with migrating myoelectric complexes (MMC). The MMC consists of three phases of activity:

- *Phase 1.* The quiescent phase. There is no spiking activity.
- *Phase 2.* Irregular contractive activity is initiated and increases in intensity.
- *Phase 3.* The dominant phase. Bursts of constant, intense intestinal contractions occur at the maximal frequency. Peristalsis of consecutive intestinal segments takes place. Propulsion of intestinal contents is at a peak and they are swept away in an aboral direction. This phase of the MMC has been aptly described as the 'gastrointestinal housekeeper'. These activity fronts migrate over a 90–120 min period from the antrum of the stomach to the terminal ileum in continuous succession.

The MMC, besides transporting digested food products, removes the mucus layer that is continuously replenished and prevents prolonged contact between enteric pathogens, toxins, and the mucosa of the intestine. Laboratory studies on rats have demonstrated that if the MMC is abolished with drugs (morphine and phenylephrine) for more than 6–15 hours, bacterial overgrowth develops. On cessation of the drugs and the return of the MMC, bacterial overgrowth is abolished. When motility decreases stasis occurs. The products of digestion are an ideal milieu for bacteria to multiply and cause diarrhoea.

The propulsive functions of the intestine are exaggerated when diarrhoea occurs. Increased fluid within the lumen increases motility and the rapid evacuation of intestinal contents prevents or minimizes contact between the mucosal surface of the intestine and the pathogens themselves or their toxins. This raises the question of the role of antimotility agents in the treatment of infective diarrhoea.

The systemic diseases and local conditions listed below involve the small intestine and decrease motility, leading to bacterial overgrowth and diarrhoea (see Chapter 9).

Causes of decreased small intestinal motility

- Diabetic autonomic neuropathy
- Hypothyroidism
- Amyloidosis
- Scleroderma
- Myotonia dystrophica (a hereditary condition characterized by myotonia, muscular wasting, cataracts, testicular atrophy and frontal baldness)
- Lymphoma
- Intestinal pseudo-obstruction
- Radiation enteritis

Drug therapy is also an important cause of decreased intestinal motility and is discussed in Chapter 7.

Mucus

A thick layer of mucus covers the epithelial surface of the intestine to protect the mucosa and lubricate the movement of digested food and faeces (in the colon). Mucus is synthesized and secreted by cells in the gastrointestinal tract. Mucus consists of 95 per cent water, interlinked glycoprotein molecules with a high carbohydrate content, small amounts of proteins and lipids, enmeshed micro-organisms, cells, cell debris, products of digestion and protein from gastrointestinal secretions.

The mucus layer protects the mucosa from enteric pathogens and bacterial toxins, antigens, dietary chemicals and injurious components of bile, pancreatic juice and intestinal secretions. The role of the mucus layer as a major physical impediment to enteric pathogens may be overstated. Mucus provides a barrier to those pathogens that adhere to the mucosa, and is a lubricant which coats pathogens to ease their removal from the gut by peristalsis. A more sophisticated form of protection by the mucus is directed against bacteria. The carbohydrate composition of the glycoprotein mimics the surface of the epithelial cell. Bacteria (which damage the cell by adherence) are thus misinformed, misled and entrapped by the mucus.

For bacteria that secrete a toxin, other preventive strategies are employed. Cholera toxin increases mucus production that binds the toxin and decreases diffusion to the intestinal mucosal cells. Another protective mechanism attributed to the mucus layer is effected by lysozyme, a protein within the mucus layer that kills bacteria.

The small intestine also prevents or minimizes injury to itself and the host by the antibacterial action of bile and pancreatic secretions. Proteolytic enzymes cause bacterial lysis and in vitro some viruses are susceptible to the action of trypsin. Further protection against injury to the mucosa by bacterial adherence occurs by the constant shedding and renewal of the enterocytes.

The ileocaecal valve

The ileocaecal valve (ICV) is another possible defence mechanism of the gastrointestinal tract. The ICV at the boundary between the small intestine and the colon regulates the passage of digested food and prevents reflux of contaminated large bowel contents to the relatively sterile small intestine. This prevents bacterial colonization of the small intestine, subsequent deconjugation of bile salts, fat malabsorption and diarrhoea. This preventive role is attributed to the ICV because bacterial colony counts in the ileal region adjacent to the ICV are significantly low compared with counts in the caecum. The functions of the ICV are still in question as ileocaecal resection does not lead to altered motility of the bowel and derangement of luminal contents, nor bacterial colonization of the small intestine.

Colonic defences

Normal bacterial flora

Although intestinal infection is minimized by the mechanisms discussed, in the elderly, due to the variety of factors mentioned, many pathogens may survive and reach the colon.

The normal bacterial flora in the colon provide a further 'line' of defence. The bacterial composition of the colon is unique to each individual and is determined early in life by interactions between the host and the bacteria, and between bacteria themselves. The number and types of colonic bacteria are relatively constant throughout life. Even a major change from a nonvegetarian to a vegetarian diet does not significantly alter the species nor the number of colonic flora.

The normal colonic bacteria resist eviction to the exterior with faeces by attaching to the colonic mucosa. 'New' pathogens cannot gain occupancy in the colon as the adhesion sites are already occupied by the commensal bacteria.

These commensal bacteria in the colon form a complex well balanced ecological system to protect the host against infection by a variety of mechanisms: modification of bile acids; stimulation of peristalsis; induction of immunological responses; depletion of essential substrates from the environment; competition for adhesion sites; creation of restrictive metabolic environments and elaboration of antibiotic-like substances. Therapy with antibiotics (see Chapter 7) affects both the pathogens for which they were intended and, unfortunately, the normal flora. In the 'ecological vacuum' that results, organisms injurious to the host, such as *Clostridium difficile,* proliferate with adverse consequences to the host (see Chapter 8).

Motility

In the colon, motility occurs through two types of waves: segmenting and propulsive. The role of colonic motility as a defence mechanism is not well established.

BIBLIOGRAPHY AND FURTHER READING

Anuras, S. & Sutherland, J. (1984). Jejunal manometry in healthy elderly subjects. *Gastroenterology* **86**:1016.

Calam, J., Goodlad, R.A., Lee, C.Y. et al. (1991). Achlorhydria-induced hypergastrinaemia: the role of bacteria. *Clin. Sci.* **80**:281–4.

Cash, R.A., Music, S.T., Libonati, J.P., Snyder M.J.J., Wenzel, R.P. & Hornick, R.B. (1974). Response of man to infection with *Vibrio cholerae.* I. Clinical, serologic and bacteriologic responses to known inoculum. *J. Infect. Dis.* **129**:45–52.

Clamp, J. (1986). The role of mucus in human intestinal defence. In *Gut Defences in Clinical Practice,* ed. M.S. Losowsky & R.V. Heatley, pp. 83–94. Edinburgh: Churchill Livingstone.

Feldman, M., Cryer, B., McArthur, K.E., Huet, B.A. & Lee, E. (1996). Effects of aging and gastritis on gastric acid and pepsin secretion in humans: a prospective study. *Gastroenterology* **110**:1043–52.

Giannella, R.A., Broitman, S.A. & Zamchek, N. (1973). Influence of gastric acidity on bacterial and parasitic enteric infections. A perspective. *Ann. Intern. Med.* **78**:271–6.

Holt, P.R. (1991). Approach to gastrointestinal problems in the elderly. In *Textbook of Gastroenterology,* Vol. 1, ed. T. Yamada, pp. 882–99. Philadelphia: Lippincott.

Hurwitz, A., Brady, D.A., Schaal, S.E., et al. (1997). Gastric acidity in older adults. *J. Am. Med. Assoc.* **278**:659–62.

Papadopolous, C., Kalantzis, N., Rekoumis, G. et al. (1985). A comparative trial of 400 mg cimetidine twice daily and 100 mg daily in the short-term treatment of duodenal ulceration. *Curr. Med. Res. Opin.* **9**:511–5.

Rahman, Q., Haboubi, N.Y., Hudson, P.R., Lee, G.S. & Shah, I.U. (1991). The effect of thyroxine on small intestinal motility in the elderly. *Clin. Endocrinol. (Oxf.)* **35**:443–6.

Rolfe, D.R. (1984). Interactions among micro-organisms of the indigenous intestinal flora and their influence on the host. *Rev. Infect. Dis.* **6**:73S–79S.

Russell, R.M. (1992). Changes in gastrointestinal function attributed to aging. *Am. J. Clin. Nutr.* **55**:1203S-1207S.

Sarker, S.A. & Gyr, K. (1992). Non-immunological defence mechanisms of the gut. *Gut* **33**:987–93.

Simon, G.L. & Gorbach, S.L. (1986). The human intestinal microflora. *Dig. Dis. Sci.* **31**:147S-162S.

Thorens, J., Froehlich, F., Schwizer, W. et al. (1996). Bacterial overgrowth during treatment with Omeprazole compared with Cimetidine: a prospective randomised double blind study. *Gut* **39**:54–9.

Walker, K.J., Gilliland, S.S., Vance-Bryan, K. et al. (1993). *Clostridium difficile* colonization in residents of long-term care facilities: prevalence and risk factors. *J. Am. Geriatr. Soc.* **41**:940–6.

Immune defences of the aging gut

R. Logan Faust

Introduction

With the development of monoclonal antibodies and molecular immunology used to study cell populations, large gains have been made in the understanding of the body's immune defence. Paralleling this is an increased interest in the effect of advancing age on susceptibility to infection, largely due to the rapidly increasing size of the geriatric population. In the USA it is estimated that the elderly occupy 90 per cent of the beds in long-term care facilities and account for nearly 50 per cent of the total health care costs. As they are the fastest growing segment of the population, their importance to the health care system will continue to increase.

The systemic immune system

Aging clearly affects the systemic immune system. Thymic involution is complete by approximately 50 years of age and the level of thymic hormone is undetectable after the age of 60. This may lead to diminished promotion of lymphocyte differentiation and a reduced ability of T cells to elicit a graft versus host response. Additionally, there is a decrease in the response of T cells to nonspecific mitogens and a decrease in the production of cytokines such as interleukin-2. These effects are due to functional alterations that occur with aging as opposed to a depletion in the absolute numbers of cells.

In the humoral arm of the systemic immune system, it is proposed that the major defect with aging is impairment of regulatory function. This is manifested by defective T helper cell activity, enhanced suppressor cell activity, or both. T cell dependent antibody response shows greater impairment with aging than does the T cell independent response. Absolute concentrations of immunoglobulins may be increased slightly in the elderly due to increased levels of IgA and IgG; however, there is an impaired generation of specific antibody following stimulation by antigen.

The gastrointestinal tract is in contact with a variety of bacterial, dietary and enzymatic antigens over an area estimated to be between 200 and 300 square metres. An immune defence localized to this tissue and functioning partly independent of the systemic immune system, was first demonstrated in the early 1900s. Epidemiological data suggest a correlation between aging, changes in the gastrointestinal tract's immune defence, and an increased incidence of, and fatality from, infectious diseases of the gastrointestinal tract. Compared with systemic immunity, there was little work until recently on the specific changes in the gastrointestinal immune system due to aging. Mitogen-induced proliferation of the lymphoid tissue in the gut immune system of mice decreases with age although at a slower rate than in the splenic cells that are representative of the systemic immune system. Additionally, the production of interleukin-2 by T cells in the Peyer's patches of the mouse gut immune system also declines with aging, but at an average age of 24 months as opposed to 21 months for the decrease seen with splenic tissue. This implies that the gut-associated lymphoid tissue has a later onset and slower rate of functional decline in certain aspects than the corresponding components of the systemic immune system.

This chapter covers the basic structure of the gastrointestinal immune system and incorporates those changes which have been shown to develop with advancing age.

Overview

The gastrointestinal immune system is a portion of the mucosa-associated lymphoid tissue (MALT). MALT provides immunity to areas that possess mucosal surfaces directly exposed to the environment. Gut-associated lymphoid tissue is spread the length of the gastrointestinal tract and its immune response is largely humoral. The predominant immunoglobulin that affects this response is IgA. Additionally, IgA is the most prevalent immunoglobulin in human intestinal secretions. In serum, IgA comprises only 10 to 15 per cent of the total immunoglobulin pool. It is secreted as a complex of two monomers joined by a polypeptide known as the J chain. In its secreted form, this dimeric IgA accounts for nearly 95 per cent of the IgA in normal intestinal fluid.

The immune system of the gut is composed of various cells, each of which performs a specialized function. Antigen reception by cells in the Peyer's patches provides the initial stimulus to B cells. The primed B cells migrate via blood and lymphatics to the lamina propria. Here, terminal differentiation to IgA-secreting plasma cells occurs. These plasma cells produce J chain-containing dimeric IgA that is then transported across the intestinal cell to be secreted into the lumen of the gut as secretory IgA (sIgA).

The enteric immune system is fully developed by two years of age. Studies of whole gut lavage fluid show no difference in the composition or total concentration of immunoglobulins between subjects 70 years of age and those aged 20 to 50 years. This corresponds to a study of cultured human duodenal mucosa in which the production of immunoglobulin was the same in young (less than or equal to 50 years) and old (greater than or equal to 70 years) subjects. Also, the level of antibody in gut fluid after exposure to the dietary proteins gliadin, ovalbumin and ß-lactoglobulin is the same in these two groups of patients.

Antigen recognition

Recognition of intestinal antigen and the initiation of the intestinal immune response take place in the Peyer's patches. These are aggregates of lymphoid cells that extend through the mucosa into the submucosa of the small intestine. Most of these are located in the terminal ileum. The number of patches increases through puberty to a peak of about 200 per intestine. From the age of 20, there is a gradual decline, to a plateau of approximately 100 in persons aged 70 to 95 years. This is not related to a change in the surface area of the small intestine, as jejunal biopsies have shown no reduction in area and no change in morphology because of aging. The lymphoid cells are grouped in the follicles, which contain mostly B cells, and interfollicular areas where the predominant cell type is the T cell bearing a CD4 cell surface marker. The number of follicles in each Peyer's patch decreases with age. A similar age-related loss of follicles occurs in the human large intestine.

The uptake of antigen by the epithelium of the Peyer's patches in the small intestine and the solitary follicles of the large intestine provides the first stimulus to lymphoid cells to begin the immune response (Figure 2.1). Antigen uptake occurs in the small intestine through a specialized follicle-associated epithelium that overlies the surface or dome of the Peyer's patches. This epithelium is relatively deficient in mucus-producing goblet cells and has no IgA transporting capacity that leaves it more accessible to contact with antigen.

Follicle-associated epithelium also contains specialized cells known as membranous or 'M' cells which lack fully developed microvilli on their surface. Via pinocytosis, these cells transport luminal antigens inward to within 0.3 mm of lymphocytes in the Peyer's patches. Thus, B cells and T cells are 'primed', the former by direct recognition of antigenic determinants on the antigen itself, and the latter by recognition of antigenic determinants in association with major histocompatibility complex molecules. There is no information concerning the function of the M cells and aging. Other phagocytic cells, however, show a variable response to aging. For example, the Küpffer cells of the liver exhibit an age-related reduction in the capacity to endocytose and process particulate antigens, while the circulating mononuclear cells are unchanged.

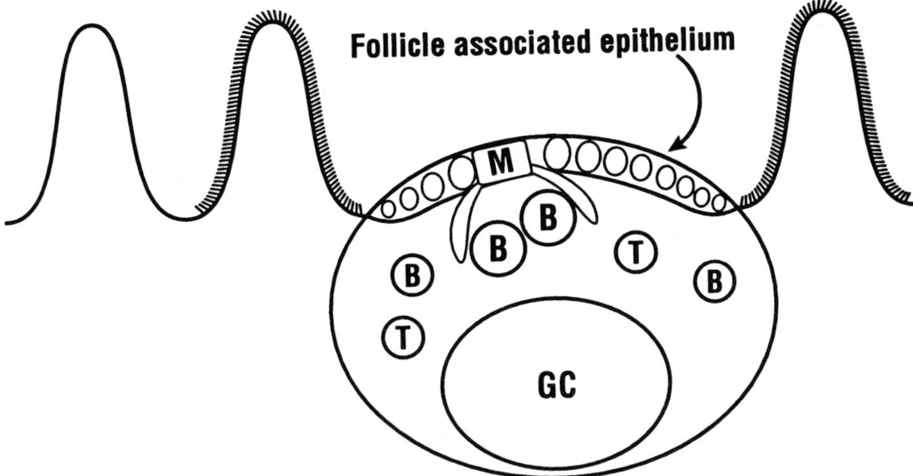

Figure 2.1.   Diagrammatic representation of a Peyer's patch with overlying follicle-associated epithelium. M cells (M) are in close proximity to immature lymphocytes (B and T) and present antigen, thereby priming the immune response. The germinal centre (GC) is also shown.

Migration and differentiation of B cells

Commitment of the B cells to the IgA class occurs predominantly in the germinal centre of the lymphoid follicle. This is regulated in an incompletely understood fashion by T lymphocytes present in Peyer's patches and, perhaps, by continual antigen-driven division in the absence of signals for further differentiation. With aging a reduction in the ratio of helper to suppressor T cells in the Peyer's patches occurs. This may explain the decline in in vitro immunoglobulin production and proliferative responses seen in aged cells from the Peyer's patches, and mesenteric lymph nodes during stimulation by T cell dependent B cell mitogens.

B cells primed in Peyer's patches do not mature into antibody-secreting plasma cells there. They leave the lymphoid follicle and travel, via mesenteric lymph nodes, to the thoracic duct and peripheral circulation (Figure 2.2). Control of B cell localization to particular tissues is mediated through antigens on the cell itself interacting with receptors in other tissues. 'Homing antigens' on the surface of immature lymphocytes interact with specific receptors called 'addressins' found on the surface of endothelial lined venules in the mesenteric and peripheral lymph nodes. This interaction leads to localization of lymphocytes to selective tissues of the common mucosal immune system. This includes not only the lamina propria and intraepithelial regions of the intestine but also such extraintestinal sites as the bronchus-associated lymphoid tissue, mammary gland and female genital tract. T lymphocyte dependent maturation and terminal differentiation then occurs yielding immunoglobulin-secreting plasma cells.

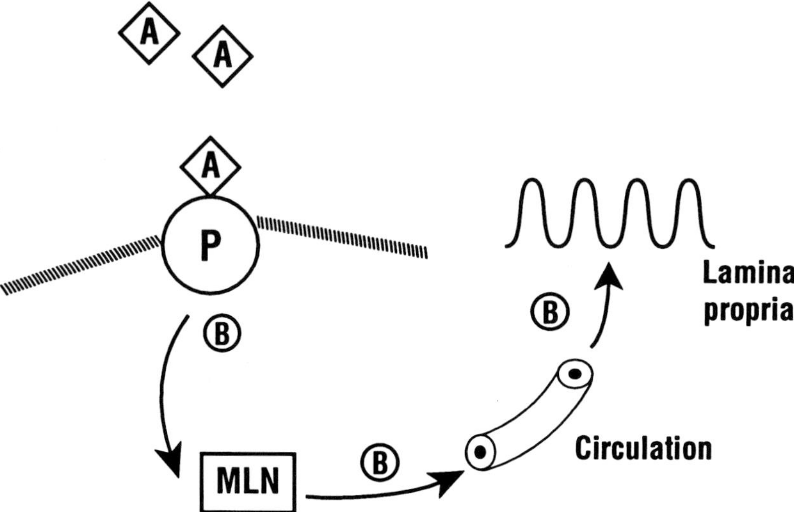

Figure 2.2.   Migration and homing of B lymphocytes. Antigen (A) is presented at the Peyer's patch (P) and primed B lymphocytes then migrate via the mesenteric lymph nodes (MLN) to the circulation and eventually to specific tissues.

The lamina propria

The lamina propria of the intestine contains B and T lymphocytes, plasma cells, macrophages, mast cells and eosinophils, all of which are presumed to have some role in the immune response. T cells of the helper type are felt to be important in the activation, growth and differentiation of the surrounding B cells, 70 to 90 per cent of which demonstrate IgA on immunofluorescent staining. Macrophages present antigen to T lymphocytes, are active in bacterial phagocytosis, and produce soluble substances such as interleukin-1 which assist with T cell activation. Mast cells may release mediators that alter vascular permeability, mucus production and the recruitment of inflammatory cells. In old (>24 month) Fischer rats there is an increased density of CD8 lymphocytes in the lamina propria of the small intestine as compared with adult rats three to six months of age. These suppressor cells may contribute to the diminished differentiation of IgA-producing plasma cells or to the local suppression of antibody production seen in older animals in this model of aging.

The nature and function of secretory IgA

Secretory IgA (sIgA) is the most important component of the defence against infectious organisms and dietary antigens produced in the gut lumen. The compound

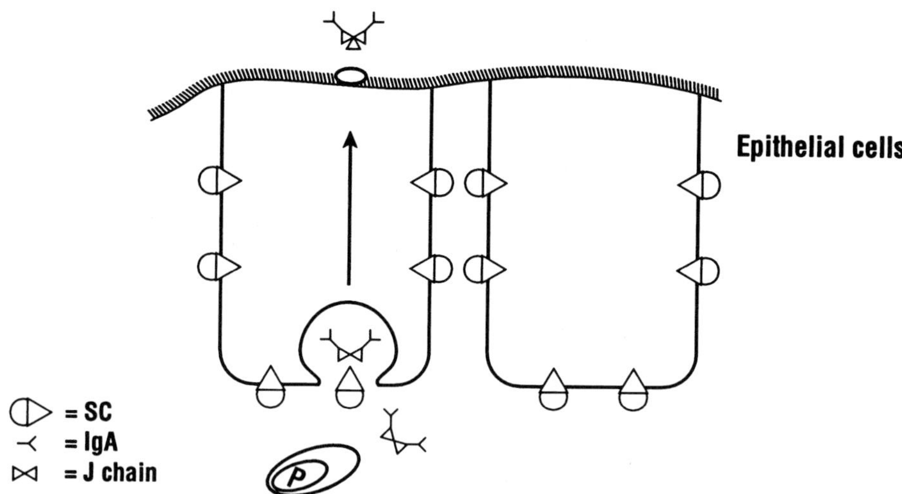

Figure 2.3.   Production and transport of sIgA. Plasma cells (P) secrete dimeric IgA that is bound to SC molecules on the basal and lateral surface of gastrointestinal epithelial cells. This complex is then transported across the cell and out into the intestinal lumen. A portion of the SC molecule remains attached to the epithelium.

is composed of two IgA monomers and two important additional polypeptides – SC, or secretory component, and the J chain. SC's importance lies in the noncovalent interaction between it and the IgA dimer that decreases the susceptibility of the antibody to dissolution on passage through the gut. J chain is essential for the external transport of dimeric IgA through the epithelial cells of the intestinal border as its incorporation creates the binding sites for the molecule to these cells.

SC is produced predominantly by columnar cells of the crypts of Lieberkuhn and is expressed on the basal and lateral surface of secretory epithelial cells that are also largely found in the crypts. It acts as the epithelial cell surface receptor with the dimeric IgA–J chain complex. Bound SC–immunoglobulin complexes are endocytosed and transported across the cell to the apical membrane where the SC molecule is proteolytically split. A portion remains bound to the apical membrane and the remainder is covalently bound to the IgA–J chain complex forming the complete sIgA molecule (Figure 2.3).

IgA is produced by B lymphocytes and plasma cells of the laminal propria, and this production marks the terminal step in the differentiation of the B lymphocyte. In mice there is a small but significant decline in the gut IgA content with aging. In the serum of both mice and humans, a slight increase is noted with age. As mentioned before, in human whole gut lavage fluid there is no difference in the concentration of IgA, IgM or IgG between subjects greater than 70 years and those less than 50 years of age.

Secretory IgA has its main function in 'immune exclusion': that is, protection of the surface of epithelial cells against dietary antigens and infectious agents. The secretory form of the immunoglobulin has a greater antibody specificity than the corresponding systemic form. This may be useful to cope with the diverse antigenic character of micro-organisms. sIgA binds directly to bacteria such as *Vibrio cholerae* and prevents their adherence to and subsequent colonization of intestinal epithelial cells. sIgA has also been reported to neutralize toxins secreted by these micro-organisms. There is even a role for sIgA in the inhibition of viral replication and mucosal invasion. Dietary antigens are also bound in the intestine, thereby limiting their absorption and, therefore, the development of serum antibodies and related immune complexes.

As in humans, in a rhesus monkey model total IgA concentration in whole gut lavage fluid is independent of age. However, antigen specific IgA antibody levels were markedly reduced in old as compared with young animals. Additionally, flow cytometry has shown that the relative number of peripheral blood lymphocytes expressing surface IgA or cholera toxin antigens after intraduodenal immunization with cholera toxin is reduced in older animals. It is suggested that the decrease in the pool of antigen specific B lymphocytes decreases the number of cells migrating back to the lamina propria of the intestine and thereby decreasing specific IgA antibody production.

Intraepithelial lymphocytes and cell-mediated cytotoxicity

A fraction of Peyer's patch cells in mice migrate to the spaces between the columnar epithelial cells which line the villi of the intestine and are termed 'intraepithelial lymphocytes'. The majority of these cells in humans are T lymphocytes – 80 to 90 per cent express the CD8 surface marker. The percentage of these cells that actually arise from Peyer's patches is unknown for man and rodents. They have been shown in rodents to mediate direct cytotoxic activities. In humans, they are prominent in the small intestinal mucosa of patients with tropical and nontropical sprue and are seen in infections such as Giardia and AIDS; however, their role has not been defined. Although small populations of cells such as natural killer and killer cells mediate cytotoxic reactions in both the intraepithelial region and the lamina propria, the possibility of T cells functioning in a similar fashion in these locations is not well demonstrated in vivo.

Malnutrition

There is no direct role of aging in the quantity of sIgA secreted in the gut of healthy persons. There is indirect evidence that diseases associated with aging may cause a change in IgA production. In severe protein–calorie malnutrition in the elderly the level of sIgA is significantly reduced when measured in tears. This deficiency could be reversed with improved nutrition. No corresponding studies looking at sIgA production in the gut have been performed.

Tolerance

Enteric antigens not only play a role in eliciting a local immune response but they also may produce some degree of systemic response. Whether enteric exposure to antigen results in priming and stimulation of the systemic immune system or to suppression of the systemic response depends on many factors. These include previous antigen exposure, health of the host, genetic background and, importantly, age.

The ability of antigens in the intestine to activate a mucosal immune response while suppressing the systemic response is the basis of oral tolerance. Suppression of the systemic immune system here may be useful to the host in two ways. First, by preventing innocuous, widespread, nonpathogenic antigens from stimulating systemic allergic reactions. Secondly, by avoiding cross-reactions with self proteins leading to autoimmune phenomena.

Tolerance induction has been studied in young and aged mice by oral administration of sheep red blood cells. Young (two-month-old) mice given sheep red blood cells orally for two weeks become tolerant to a subsequent systemic sheep red blood cell challenge. However, older (one year) mice resisted tolerance induction and produced a prominent systemic IgA response. This implies that the tolerance-inducing function of the gut-associated lymphoid tissue declines with age. This may partially explain the increase in autoimmune markers noted in the elderly as reactions to denatured self proteins.

Other studies in mice have shown that tolerance induction is reliant on the suppressor T cell. In these studies, hyporesponsiveness of the T suppressor cell is noted in senescent animals and this leads to hyperreactive systemic humoral responses to noninvasive microbial enteric antigens. This diminished T cell response could be partially corrected by exogenous interleukin-2 administration.

Clearly, the gastrointestinal immune system is a complex aggregation of numerous cells and soluble factors. Humoral defence appears to predominate but it should be borne in mind that little is known concerning the effect of the T lymphocyte and cell-mediated immunity in the gut. In this chapter aging is shown to affect many different aspects of the gastrointestinal immune system such as tolerance, antigen specific antibody production, proliferation of lymphoid tissue, and cell subset compositions and interactions. It is perhaps these changes that explain the increase in infections and tumours seen with advancing age. The developing interest in diseases of the elderly promises much in the way of future progress.

BIBLIOGRAPHY AND FURTHER READING

Ajitsu, S., Mirabella, S. & Kawanishi, H. (1990). In vivo immunologic intervention in age-related T cell defects in murine gut-associated lymphoid tissues by IL 2. *Mech. Ageing Dev.* 54:163–83.

Arranz, E., O'Mahony, S., Barton, J.R. & Ferguson, A. (1992). Immunosenescence and mucosal immunity: significant effects of old age on secretory IgA concentrations and intraepithelial lymphocyte counts. *Gut* 33:882–6.

Brandtzaeg, P., Baklien, K., Bjerke, K. et al. (1987). Nature and properties of the human gastrointestinal immune system. In *Immunology of the Gastrointestinal Tract*, Vol. I, ed. K. Miller & S. Nicklin, pp 1–85. Boca Raton, Boston: CRC Press Inc.

Butcher, E.C., Rouse, R.V., Coffman, R.L. et al. (1982). Surface phenotype of Peyer's patch germinal centre cells: implications for the role of germinal centres in B cell differentiation. *J. Immunol* 129:2698–707.

Corazza, G.R., Frazzoni, M., Gatto, M.R. & Gasbarrini, G. (1986). Aging and small bowel mucosa: a morphometric study. *Gerontology* 32:60–5.

Cornes, J.S. (1965). Number, size, and distribution of Peyer's patches in the human small intestine. *Gut* 6:225–9.

Daniels, C.K., Perez, P. & Schmucker, D.L. (1993). Alterations in CD8[+] cell distribution in gut-associated lymphoid tissues (GALT) of the aging Fischer 344 rat: a correlated immunohistochemical and flow cytometric analysis. *Exp. Gerontol.* 28:549–55.

Gallatin, W.M., Weissman, I.L. & Butcher, E.C. (1983). A cell surface molecule involved in organ-specific homing of lymphocytes. *Nature* 304:30–4.

Hosokawa, T., Motoi, S., Aoike, A. et al. (1988). Effect of aging on immunological memory in gastrointestinal tract induced by sheep red blood cells in mice. *Gastroenterologia Japonica* 23:13–17.

Kagnoff, M.F. (1993). Immunology and inflammation of the gastrointestinal tract. In *Gastrointestinal Disease: Pathophysiology, Diagnosis, Management*, ed. M.H. Sleisenger & J.S. Fordtran, pp. 45–86. Philadelphia: Saunders.

Kawanishi, H. (1993). Recent progress in senescence-associated gut mucosal immunity. *Dig. Dis.* 11:157–72.

Kawanishi, H., Ajitsu, S. & Mirabella, S. (1990). Impaired humoral immune responses to mycobacterial antigen in aged murine gut-associated lymphoid tissues. *Mech. Ageing Dev.* 54:143–61.

Koyama, K., Hosokawa, T. & Aoike, A. (1990). Aging effect on the immune functions of murine gut-associated lymphoid tissues. *Dev. Comp. Immunol.* 14:465–73.

Penn, M.D., Purkins, L., Kelleher, J., Heatley, R.V. & Mascie-Taylor, B.H. (1991). Ageing and duodenal mucosal immunity. *Age Aging* 20:33–6.

Saltzman, R.L. & Peterson, P.K. (1987). Immunodeficiency of the elderly. *Rev. Infect. Dis.* 9:1127–39.

Schmucker, D.L. & Daniels, C.K. (1986). Aging, gastrointestinal infections, and mucosal immunity. *J. Am. Geriatr. Soc.* 34:377–84.

Taylor, L.D., Daniels, C.K. & Schmucker, D.L. (1992). Ageing compromises gastrointestinal mucosal immune response in the rhesus monkey. *Immunology* 75:614–18.

Tseng, J. (1984). A population of resting IgM-IgD double-bearing lymphocytes in Peyer's patches: the major precursor cells for IgA plasma cells in the gut lamina propria. *J. Immunol.* 132:2730–5.

Udall, J.N., Pang, K., Fritze, L., Kleinman, R. & Walker, W.A. (1981). Development of gastrointestinal mucosal barrier. I. The effect of age on intestinal permeability to macromolecules. *Pediatr. Res.* 15:241–4.

Watson, R.R., McMurray, D.N., Martin, P. & Reyes, M.A. (1985). Effect of age, malnutrition, and renutrition on free secretory component and IgA in secretion. *Am. J. Clin. Nutr.* 42:281–8.

Part II

Diarrhoea

3   Pathophysiology of diarrhoea

Ranjit N. Ratnaike

In a healthy individual the frequency of bowel actions varies from three motions a day to three per week. Diarrhoea is defined as three or more unformed bowel actions in 24 hours, although this definition should not be used rigidly. Diarrhoea is also defined in terms of stool weight. Since the bulk of stool consists of water, stool weight reflects water content. In normal subjects on a western diet, the stool weight is less than 200 g/day.

In an elderly patient with a long history of constipation, a change in bowel habit to one or two loose motions warrants inquiry.

This chapter discusses the intestinal absorption and secretion of electrolytes and fluids, the regulatory processes, causes of derangement and the mechanisms of diarrhoea.

Absorption and secretion

In the gastrointestinal tract absorption and secretion of water and electrolytes occur continuously to maintain homeostasis of body fluids. Approximately 90 per cent of fluids from dietary sources, salivary, gastric, small intestinal, pancreatic and biliary secretions that amount to ten litres per day, is reabsorbed by the intestine. Most of the fluid is absorbed in the jejunum which has the largest surface area. A lesser quantity, three to five litres, is absorbed by the ileum. The colon absorbs the remainder of one to two litres but, due to its reserve capacity, can absorb up to five litres. Depending on the type of food ingested the luminal contents of the duodenum may be hypertonic or hypotonic in relation to plasma. Major fluxes of ions and fluid take place to ensure that the luminal contents are isotonic when the jejunum is reached.

Water and electrolyte absorption is by the epithelial cells (enterocytes) of the intestine (Figure 3.1), while secretion is a crypt cell activity. Water absorption is a passive process due to active electrolyte transport, especially Na, by the intestinal epithelial cells. Electroneutral Na and Cl absorption occurs primarily in the small intestine as one of three different cotransport mechanisms that effect equal molar

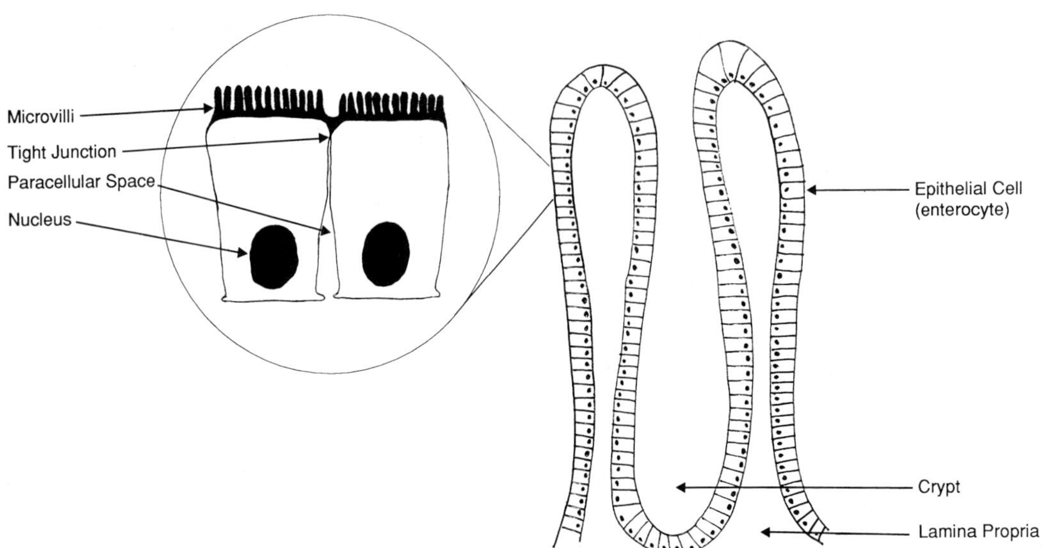

Figure 3.1.   Schematic diagram of intestinal villi and enterocytes.

absorption of Na and Cl ions. In the colon, Na and Cl absorption is predominantly an electrogenic process where Na enters the epithelial cell due to the low potential difference created in the cell by the Na–K exchange pump.

The Na–K exchange pump is one of three monovalent pumps in the intestine (the others are the calcium pump and the K–H_2 pump in the colon). It is located in the basolateral membrane of the epithelial cell. The Na–K exchange pump moves three Na ions out of the cell in exchange for two K ions. The energy for this activity is derived from the hydrolysis of one molecule of ATP by ATPase. Ultimately a potential difference of about 35–40 mV exists across the epithelial cell membrane. This provides an electrochemical gradient for the (electrogenic) entry of Na and water from the intestinal lumen into the cell.

To a lesser extent, the entry of water and electrolytes (and small molecules) from the lumen of the intestine occurs paracellularly through the tight junction in response to existing transepithelial gradients. The tight junction is present between epithelial cells and separates the paracellular space and the contents of the intestinal lumen (Figure 3.1).

In the colon further absorption occurs. The right side of the colon (embryologically distinct from the left side) is the major site of absorption. The conversion of fluid intestinal contents to faeces begins; both Na and water are avidly absorbed. The concentration of poorly absorbed ions such as Mg, Ca, PO_4 and SO_4, if present, is increased due to fluid absorption. At a sufficiently high luminal concentration these ions act as osmotic agents and their role in the pathogenesis of diarrhoea is discussed later in this chapter.

Secretion takes place in the crypt cells of both the small intestine and the colon. The major organ of secretion is the small intestine and its capacity to secrete fluid parallels its vast absorptive capacity. In patients infected with *Vibrio cholerae*, cholera toxin acts on the small intestine to cause fluid losses of up to 15 litres in a single day.

The mechanism of action of cholera toxin-like compounds, termed secretagogues (secretory agents), is described later in this chapter. If secretagogues cause intestinal secretion that overwhelms absorption, diarrhoea results.

Mechanisms of diarrhoea

The basic mechanisms that cause diarrhoea are few despite many aetiological factors. In the normal small and large intestine, absorption is the net result of active secretion and absorption of electrolytes and water. Diarrhoea occurs when the absorptive capacity of the intestine is exceeded. This may result from excessive secretion in the presence of normal absorption. Or, despite normal secretion, decreased absorption may occur, for example due to diffuse mucosal disease of the small intestine or decreased surface area of the intestine due to surgical excision. Despite vast luminal increases in fluid and electrolytes, diarrhoea will occur only if the absorptive capacity of the intestine, mainly the colon, is exceeded.

Secretory diarrhoea

Secretory diarrhoea occurs when the balance between secretion and absorption is deranged due to an increase in intracellular cyclic nucleotides, cyclic AMP or, less commonly, cyclic GMP by a secretagogue. In other instances secretory activity is mediated by an intracellular increase in calcium.

Secretory diarrhoea is the culmination of a series of complex intracellular events (Box 3.1). The process is exemplified by the action of cholera toxin (Box 3.2). The initial event is the binding of the toxin to a receptor site on the cell surface. Then, through a series of steps adenylate cyclase is activated. Adenylate cyclase reacts with ATP to generate cyclic AMP, which then activates a protein kinase that phosphorylates membrane proteins involved in active ion transport. The outcome is an increased secretion of Cl (predominantly) and HCO_3 by the crypt cells, and decreased electroneutral Na and Cl and water absorption by the more mature intestinal epithelial cells of the villi. Increased secretory activity primarily occurs in the small intestine and rarely in the colon. In summary, a secretagogue acts to 'switch' the intestinal epithelial cells from a state of net absorption to net secretion. The mechanism is a series of *biochemical* intracellular events.

Secretory diarrhoea is voluminous and unaffected by fasting. The intestinal mucosa is normal and blood in the faeces is not a feature. The stool osmolality parallels the plasma osmolality with no osmotic gap (see Chapter 5).

Box 3.1. The process of activation and deactivation of adenylate cyclase

How does a secretagogue and its receptor activate adenylate cyclase?

Preliminary information
The activation process involves two intermediaries:
1. The Gs protein.
2. Guanosine triphosphate (GTP) or guanosine diphosphate (GDP).
The Gs protein is a peripheral membrane protein consisting of three subunits (α, β, γ subunits). The Gs protein can bind to either GTP or GDP. The Gs protein–GTP complex *activates* adenylate cyclase. The Gs protein–GDP complex *inhibits* adenylate cyclase.

The process of activation
When a secretagogue binds to its receptor the following events occur:

- The Gs protein binds to GTP by the α subunit as shown:

$$\alpha\beta\gamma + \text{GTP} \xrightarrow{\text{GTPase}} \alpha\text{-GTP} + \beta\gamma$$

- α-GTP now activates adenylate cyclase which, in turn, forms cyclic adenosine monophosphate (c-AMP) from adenosine triphosphate (ATP).

$$\text{ATP} \xrightarrow{\text{adenylate cyclase}} \text{c-AMP}$$

- Cyclic AMP activates specific protein kinases that will bring about specific physiological responses.

How is adenylate cyclase deactivated?

- The α-GTP is slowly hydrolysed to α-GDP and reforms the inactive protein GDP as shown:

$$\alpha\text{-GTP} \xrightarrow[P_i]{} \alpha\text{-GDP} \xrightarrow[\beta\gamma]{} \alpha\beta\gamma\text{-GTP} \quad (\text{inactive protein–GDP})$$

Several secretagogues cause diarrhoea. A broad classification of the common secretagogues are: bacterial enterotoxins, therapeutic agents, neurohumoral agents, and endogenous compounds. Examples of secretagogues which belong to each of these groups are listed below:

Bacterial enterotoxins

- *Vibrio cholerae*
- *Escherichia coli*
- *Staphylococcus aureus*
- Shigella sp.

Box 3.2. Mechanism of action of cholera toxin

How does cholera toxin act?

- The cholera toxin consists of an A subunit and five B subunits.
- The toxin enters intestinal mucosal cells and attaches to the Gs protein.
- Part of the A subunit of cholera toxin reacts and modifies the Gs protein by ribosylation. This involves the transfer of an ADP–ribose unit from NAD to a specific arginine on the α-G protein.
- This ribosylated complex is now unable to hydrolyse bound GTP to GDP and is locked in the active form.
- Adenylate cyclase is therefore persistently activated and cyclic AMP concentrations are consequently high.
- Specific protein kinases are activated which will stimulate the active transport of ions leading to watery diarrhoea.

- *Bacillus cereus*
- *Clostridium perfringens.*

Therapeutic agents

- Anthraquinone cathartics
- Bisacodyl
- Dioctyl sodium sulfosuccinate
- Castor oil
- Ricinoleic acid
- Phenolphthalein
- Senna
- Misoprostol.

Humoral agents

- Vasoactive intestinal peptide (VIP)
- Glucagon
- Secretin
- Calcitonin
- Bradykinin.

Endogenous agents

- Long-chain fatty acids
- Dihydroxy bile acids.

Most secretory diarrhoea is due to bacterial toxins (see Chapter 8) or, less often, a therapeutic agent (see Chapter 7). The endogenous compounds are unique in that their secretory activity occurs in the colon and not the small intestine, the usual site of secretagogue action.

Osmotic diarrhoea

Osmotic diarrhoea is another major mechanism by which diarrhoea occurs. The causative agents are osmotically active compounds that are poorly absorbed, or not absorbed at all, in the colon and are therefore present in the lumen in a high concentration. Their osmotic effect causes fluid to flow into the lumen. When the absorptive capacity of the colon is exceeded, diarrhoea occurs.

The process is physiological. No alterations occur in either the intracellular mechanisms of secretion or absorption as in secretory diarrhoea. The epithelial cells are undamaged. Osmotic diarrhoea is characterized by cessation with fasting since the osmotic load will then no longer be present in the colon.

The common osmotic agents are lactulose, sorbitol, magnesium-containing antacids, magnesium sulphate (Epsom salts), and sodium sulphate (Glauber's salt). Osmotic diarrhoea occurs secondary to *maldigestion* in pancreatic insufficiency, monosaccharide and disaccharide intolerance; and as a result of *malabsorption* in conditions of small bowel mucosal damage, for example in coeliac disease (see Chapter 11) and tropical sprue (see Chapter 9). Osmotic diarrhoea can also be caused by the overindulgence of fruit and vegetables. The excessive load of long-chain carbohydrates are not completely digested in the small intestine and undergo bacterial degradation in the colon to short-chain compounds (e.g. hydrophilic solutes) which cause an osmotic diarrhoea.

A laboratory diagnosis of osmotic diarrhoea is made when the stool osmotic gap is greater than 50 mmol per kg (see Chapter 5).

Intestinal motility

The role of intestinal motility as a mechanism of diarrhoea needs further study. Motility affects intestinal absorption: decreased motility prolongs water and electrolyte absorption; increased motility decreases intestinal absorption and may lead to diarrhoea. Motility disorders may indirectly cause diarrhoea through intestinal stasis and bacterial overgrowth (see Chapter 9).

Many diarrhoeal entities are associated with altered motility but there is as yet no substantial evidence that a causal relationship exists between intrinsic abnormalities in motility and diarrhoea.

Multiple mechanisms

In many diseases the mechanism of diarrhoea is multifactorial. Both pathophysiological processes of diarrhoea, secretory and osmotic, may operate, with one dominant.

Box 3.3. The process of toxin-induced cell death

How does a toxin destroy a cell?

The toxin forms a receptor–toxin complex before entering the cell (endocytosis).

The toxin diffuses into the cytosol.

The toxin then catalyses the transfer of the ADP ribosyl moiety to the peptide chain elongation factor 2 (EF-2).

The ribosylated EF-2 is now inactivated and unable to synthesize protein.

Cell death eventually occurs.

The mechanism of diarrhoea in inflammatory bowel disease (IBD) (see Chapter 12) is complex and possibly involves several processes. Inflammatory mediators are important in the mechanism of diarrhoea in IBD. These inflammatory mediators are produced by damage to mast cells, macrophages, eosinophils and neutrophils, and serve as powerful secretagogues. Inflammatory mediators with secretagogue activity are:

- Prostaglandin E_2
- Adenosine
- Cytokines
- Bradykinin
- Histamine
- Platelet activating factor
- Serotonin.

The cellular events leading to secretion differ. Prostaglandin E_2 increases the intracellular content of cyclic AMP while bradykinin increases the cytosolic Ca of the cell. This results in increased elevation of Cl and HCO_3 ions and the decreased passive absorption of Na, Cl and water

Inflammation is the major response when enteric pathogens cause cell injury by cytotoxin production or cell invasion. Cell invasion, intracellular multiplication of the bacteria and spread to adjacent cells, and toxin production, result in cell death (Box 3.3) and the formation of a micro-ulcer or micro-abscess. In the lamina propria the inflammatory reaction releases inflammatory mediators, which act on epithelial cells to cause diarrhoea as described above.

Inflammatory processes in the intestine, in addition to intracellular changes, contribute to diarrhoea by altering intestinal motility. Also, the exudation of blood and pus may act as osmotic solutes to initiate an osmotic type of diarrhoea.

There is still much to be understood about the precise mechanisms causing diarrhoea. It is established that increased Cl secretion in secretory diarrhoea is due to the opening up of Cl channels in the cell. Electroneutral Na and Cl absorption in the small intestine is inhibited by secretagogues, although the details of this and other processes that concurrently decrease water and electrolyte absorption by the epithelial cell need to be clarified.

Intestinal secretion and absorption are influenced by factors other than the luminal contents of the gastrointestinal tract. Attention is now focused on the enteric nervous system and its role in the pathophysiology of diarrhoea. In many mammalian species, α_2 adrenergic receptors have been identified in enterocytes. Norepinephrine acts via α_2 adrenergic receptors to inhibit adenylate cyclase activity and decrease intracellular Ca concentration. These events effect net absorption of electrolytes and fluids.

Possibly, other processes yet to be established could contribute to the pathophysiology of diarrhoea. Further understanding of the role of both the enteric nervous system and the many specialized cells with exquisitely individual functions within the intestine will advance our knowledge on the pathophysiology of diarrhoea. These advances would help in the development of affordable measures in the prevention and treatment of diarrhoea, a global problem, particularly in the developing areas of the world.

BIBLIOGRAPHY AND FURTHER READING

Barrett, K. & Dharmsathaphorn, K. (1991). Secretion and absorption: small intestine and colon. In *Textbook of Gastroenterology*, vol 1, ed. T. Yamada, pp. 265–94. Philadelphia: Lippincott.

Binder, H.J. (1991). Nutrient-induced diarrhoea. In *Diarrhoeal Diseases*, ed. M. Field, pp. 159–72. New York: Elsevier.

Chang, E.B. & Rao, M.C. (1991). Intracellular mediators of intestinal electrolyte transport. In *Diarrhoeal Diseases*, ed. M. Field, pp. 49–72. New York: Elsevier.

Corazza, G.R., Frozzoni, M., Gatto, M.R.A. & Gasbarriri, G. (1986). Ageing and small bowel mucosa: a morphometric study. *Gerontology* 32:60–5.

Field, M. (1991). Intestinal ion transport mechanisms. In *Diarrhoeal Diseases*, ed. M. Field, pp. 3–21. New York: Elsevier.

Fordtran, J.S. (1967). Speculations on the pathogenesis of diarrhoea. *Fed Proc.* 26:1405–14.

Powell, D.W. (1991). Approach to the patient with diarrhoea. In *Textbook of Gastroenterology*, vol 1, ed. T. Yamada, pp. 732–78. Philadelphia: Lippincott.

Schron, C.M. & Gianella, R.A. (1991) Bacterial enterotoxins. In *Diarrhoeal Diseases*, ed. M. Field, pp. 115–38. New York: Elsevier.

History and physical examination

Ranjit N. Ratnaike

Introduction

A well taken history and careful physical examination provide substantial information to establish a working diagnosis. History taking from an elderly patient is more difficult as compared with younger adult patients. A thorough medical evaluation is complicated and time consuming in the elderly patient who has a longer history of illness and many associated medical problems.

At the initial stage of the clinical interview there is much to be gained by establishing:

- the patient's normal bowel habit
- what is meant by diarrhoea
- whether the problem is spurious (overflow) diarrhoea due to constipation
- whether there is faecal incontinence.

Clinicians are aware that history taking is an art and not a science, and obtaining a comprehensive history is what distinguishes the competent clinician. A poor historian is more often the physician and not the patient. In the elderly history taking is more tedious and may tax the physician's patience. The dulling of memory and the propensity in old age to remember distant past events with greater clarity than recent events may pose problems. More important events, in the view of the elderly patient, have occupied the forefront of the memory stores and crowded out the less important. The recall of names and dosages of medication important to the physician may be burdensome to the patient.

In taking a history from an elderly patient, changes in style and tempo are necessary. The medical interview may be tiring to the elderly patient. Concomitant illnesses and the side-effects of medications often sap the vitality of the patient. Besides failing memory and cognition, poor hearing makes verbal communication difficult. Depression and a memory deficit are additional common barriers to obtaining information. Denial or minimizing the problem of diarrhoea, especially faecal incontinence, is not uncommon. Constipation may be regarded as 'normal'.

The time frame for obtaining a history from an elderly patient should be expanded and should ideally be flexible. History taking should be leisurely; questions repeated and clarified; the patient's memory jogged with clues, and leading questions asked; silences and requests to repeat questions accepted graciously. Importantly, the elderly patient must be allowed adequate time to reflect and recall. The pace of the interview should be set by the patient and not the physician.

Impatience, disguised and compensated for in polite verbiage, is invariably transparent and alienates most patients. The elderly patient who has good hearing, good eyesight and is cognitively intact will pick up cues, verbal or nonverbal, that reflect haste and annoyance and will respond accordingly.

An inadequate history carries with it the danger of reaching a diagnosis or hypothesis based not on fact but a 'gut feeling' or a 'hunch'. Investigations to confirm or exclude an unreasoned diagnosis or hypothesis are tedious to the patient and ethically and fiscally irresponsible.

Elderly patients, particularly those with dementia, are unreliable historians. Information should then be sought from a relative or care-giver to clarify specific issues or to obtain the entire history. The presence of a relative at the interview could result in the patient being ignored. This must be guarded against.

Onset and duration

The duration of diarrhoea has implications regarding aetiology. Acute diarrhoea is of less than two weeks' duration and most episodes settle within a few days. Although frequent causes of acute diarrhoea are dietary indiscretions, excessive alcohol ingestion or a nonspecific side-effect of medication, the most common cause is a viral or bacterial pathogen (see Chapter 8).

A viral diarrhoea, such as a Rotavirus infection (see Chapter 8), is suggested by low grade fever, vomiting, myalgia, malaise, headache and contact with a very young child with diarrhoea. Diarrhoea due to food poisoning (see Chapter 8) has a sudden onset, and vomiting is a prominent feature. The diagnosis of food-borne illness is strengthened by the clustering of cases. The onset of diarrhoea may be associated with a particular type of food. Specific bacteria often contaminate a particular type of food: *Bacillus cereus* and fried rice; *Vibrio parahaemolyticus* and sea food; enterohaemorrhagic *E. coli* 0156:H7 with minced beef in fast foods; *Campylobacter jejuni* with poultry; *Trichinella spiralis* and pork.

If the diarrhoea is chronic (over three weeks' duration), the most useful approach is to decide if the small or large intestine is involved. Specific distinguishing features are discussed subsequently in this chapter. Chronic small bowel diarrhoea is most often due to malabsorption. The bowel actions are large, frothy and foul smelling, and difficult to flush. Large bowel diarrhoea may be associated with the passage of blood and mucus.

Temporal profile

The time when diarrhoea occurs may provide diagnostic clues. Nocturnal diarrhoea always reflects pathology and is common in patients with diabetes mellitus and autonomic neuropathy. Early morning diarrhoea, usually two to three motions, is a feature of the irritable bowel syndrome. Diarrhoea soon after a meal occurs with the dumping syndrome and in some patients with amoebic colitis, and after a meal with a high fat content in coeliac disease or pancreatic disease.

Past medical history

The common drug-related (see Chapter 7) and other iatrogenic causes of diarrhoea should be considered. Diarrhoea is a feature of upper gastrointestinal surgery for peptic ulceration, resections of the intestines, especially the terminal ileum and colon, intestinal bypass procedures, pancreatic resection, and radiation therapy (see Chapter 15). A history of diarrhoea in childhood and failure to thrive points to a malabsorption syndrome such as coeliac disease (see Chapter 11). Intolerance to milk and milk products suggests lactose intolerance (see Chapter 15).

Current medical problems

Awareness of the current medical conditions for which the patient is receiving treatment is essential. This provides information on systemic diseases that may involve the gastrointestinal tract and cause diarrhoea, and medications with diarrhoea as a side-effect (see Chapter 7). Information on the patient's sexual preference is important. Patients with AIDS (see Chapter 9) and those on immunosuppressive agents are predisposed to less commonly identified pathogens, and the microbiology laboratory could then be alerted to screen for organisms not sought routinely.

Drug history

Information on what medications the patient is taking is an essential part of the clinical interview and should include a list of:

- proprietary drugs
- nonproprietary drugs
- over-the-counter medications
- purchases from health food stores, not considered drugs.

A history of diarrhoea that ceases with fasting suggests osmotic diarrhoea (see Chapters 3 and 5). Osmotic diarrhoea is usually due to a drug or dietary agent such as lactose in subjects with lactose intolerance (see Chapter 15). The possibility of laxative abuse must not be disregarded in a patient with chronic diarrhoea of elusive aetiology, however reasonable and well adjusted the patient may appear (see Chapter 7).

Psychosocial history

It is important to inquire about life events likely to act as psychosocial stressors. Prominent among these are a recent bereavement, separation, divorce, relationship problems and financial difficulties. This information may not be revealed at the first interview. However, pursuing aspects of depression or anxiety is important, especially if the irritable bowel syndrome is suspected (see Chapter 14).

Family history

A family history of diarrhoea is associated with medullary carcinoma of the thyroid (Chapter 15), and coeliac disease (see Chapter 11).

Travel abroad

Acute diarrhoea acquired during travel to the tropics or to areas of suboptimal hygiene is invariably infective in nature (see Chapter 9). A history of travel abroad, especially to areas with pathogens known to cause diarrhoea, such as *Giardia lamblia* in St. Petersburg, Russia, is important. Chronic diarrhoea after a visit to tropical and subtropical regions raises the possibility of parasitic causes (see Chapter 8), most importantly of *G. lamblia*. Inadequately treated parasitic infections can lead to chronicity or intermittent diarrhoea.

Dietary history

A dietary history is valuable in patients with chronic diarrhoea. Diarrhoea and abdominal discomfort with the ingestion of wheat products suggests coeliac disease (see Chapter 11). Diarrhoea, abdominal discomfort, borborygmi and flatulence with milk products, except yoghurt, is usually diagnostic of lactose intolerance (see Chapter 15). Patients with malabsorption either due to small bowel or pancreatic pathology complain of diarrhoea after a meal with a high fat content.

Elderly subjects may develop diarrhoea through changes to their diet. During history taking it is useful to inquire if the elderly patient has made recent dietary changes to overcome constipation, lose weight, reduce cholesterol, or adopt a healthier lifestyle.

Nausea and vomiting

Nausea and vomiting occur with viral infections, and with bacterial infections with preformed toxins, as in food poisoning. Confusion often arises when vomiting is associated with symptoms and signs of dysentery (tenesmus, diarrhoea with blood and mucus) in Shigella. The vomiting is due to the toxin secreted by the organism being absorbed during its passage through the small intestine.

Bowel actions

Many elderly patients with poor vision, problems of recall or disinterest, are unable to describe their stools. If the diarrhoeal motions are black then, in addition to melaena, the other causes of black motions should be considered:

- iron
- charcoal
- bismuth compounds
- liquorice
- blackberries.

Viewing a sample of diarrhoeal stool is always helpful.

In malabsorptive states due to a small intestinal mucosal disease or a pancreatic cause, the bowel motions are of large volume, frothy, greasy, porridge-like and are difficult to flush; there is often a film of oil in the pan. The stools are remarkably and distressingly foul smelling, a fact which would be noted by the patient and others who share the same toilet. Stools float in the pan due to their air content, not fat, and are not a pointer to malabsorption.

The presence of undigested food suggests intestinal hurry and may occur with the irritable bowel syndrome, but is not usually a feature of a malabsorptive condition. Stools which resemble rabbit droppings are frequently described by patients with the irritable bowel syndrome.

Blood and mucus

The presence of blood in the stool requires careful clarification lest both patient and physician are confused. If diarrhoea is associated with bleeding it should be established whether this is due to internal or external haemorrhoids, rectal tears, or fissures. Diarrhoea due to small intestinal pathology is not associated with blood. The presence of blood, due to haemorrhoids or a rectal tear, may incorrectly steer the diagnosis away from a small intestinal cause of diarrhoea. The most important causes of bloody diarrhoea are colonic malignancy, inflammatory bowel disease, and bacterial or protozoan infections of the colon.

Mucus secretion is an important feature of large bowel diarrhoea. Excessive mucus secretion is the hallmark of a villous adenoma.

Abdominal pain

Peri-umbilical and right lower quadrant pain is characteristic of small intestinal disease. Epigastric pain, with radiation to the back, is a feature of pancreatic malignancy and pancreatitis. The clinical picture of a peptic ulcer, and diarrhoea suggesting steatorrhoea, must alert the clinician to exclude the Zollinger–Ellison syndrome.

Iliac fossa pain or discomfort, rectal pain and tenesmus are symptoms of colonic disease. Tenesmus is described as spasms of the rectum accompanied by a desire to defaecate with no outcome. This uncomfortable and frustrating symptom, once experienced, is rarely forgotten.

Flatulence

Flatulence occurs with the irritable bowel syndrome, lactose intolerance and malabsorption, although the most common cause is air swallowing.

Systemic features

In the elderly, especially those undernourished, severe diarrhoea of even a few days with anorexia, nausea and vomiting leads to loss of weight. Significant weight loss should raise the possibility of malignancy, malabsorption, inflammatory bowel disease, thyrotoxicosis or laxative abuse.

Fever may accompany acute viral or bacterial diarrhoea. In the elderly the presence of fever with bloody diarrhoea and mucus suggests a bacteraemia associated with an invasive pathogen. Fever occurs in chronic diarrhoea due to tuberculosis (see Chapter 8), Whipple's disease (see Chapter 9), some parasitic infections (see Chapter 8) and inflammatory bowel disease (see Chapter 12).

Physical examination

Although the most valuable information is obtained from an exhaustive history, the physical examination provides additional data to formulate a confident diagnosis.

In patients, especially those with chronic diarrhoea, physical examination may be clouded by complications such as: weight loss and anaemia due to blood loss from a colonic malignancy; bone fractures due to secondary metastatic deposits or osteomalacia; oedema because of hypoalbuminemia; and bleeding diatheses due to malabsorption of vitamin K. Lymphadenopathy should be sought, especially in the left supraclavicular fossa, for metastatic evidence of an abdominal malignancy.

The skin lesions of mucosal ulceration, pyoderma gangrenosum and erythema nodosum point to inflammatory bowel disease while the presence of fistulas and anal tags specifically suggest Crohn's disease. The skin lesions of dermatitis herpetiformi, associated with coeliac disease (see Chapter 11) are intensely pruritic vesicles symmetrically distributed on the extensor surfaces of the limbs. Hyperpigmentation occurs in Whipple's disease (see Chapter 9). Taut skin over the fingers that limits extension, telangiectasia and areas of depigmentation are suspicious of scleroderma.

Musculoskeletal changes secondary to diarrhoea are unusual in the elderly. Peripheral and axial joint problems are associated with inflammatory bowel disease (see Chapter 12). In Whipple's disease peripheral, rather than axial joint involvement occurs (see Chapter 15). Patients with HLA-B27 haplotype infected with *Salmonella* sp., *Yersinia enterocolitica* and *Shigella* sp. are predisposed to Reiter's syndrome which consists of the clinical triad of arthritis, urethritis and conjunctivitis. However, this manifestation is uncommon in the elderly.

In patients with inflammatory bowel disease, especially Crohn's disease, a single or multiple peripheral joint may be swollen and painful. Ankylosing spondylitis is seen more often in ulcerative colitis and in patients with the HLA-B27 haplotype; there is a male predominance.

The abdomen may be distended due to gas or ascites. Ascites can occur in tuberculosis (see Chapter 8), a malignancy or if hypoalbuminaemia is present. Abdominal distension in an acutely ill patient with inflammatory bowel disease requires the exclusion of a toxic megacolon.

In normal subjects the sigmoid colon is palpable and mild tenderness is not unusual. In patients with the irritable bowel syndrome the colon may be markedly tender in many areas. Abdominal palpation may reveal a mass suggesting a malignancy or Crohn's disease, and in the appropriate clinical setting an amoeboma should be considered. A 'doughy' feeling on palpation due to oedematous intestines occurs in patients with intestinal tuberculosis and typhoid fever. An enlarged nodular liver suggests metastases.

A rectal examination in the elderly is mandatory and should be preceded by inspection of the perianal area for abscesses, fissures, fistulas and skin tags. On rectal examination the presence of mucus and/or blood suggests large bowel pathology. In approximately 90 per cent of cases with carcinoma of the rectum an abnormality can be felt on digital examination. Haemorrhoids should be ruled out by using a proctoscope and not a sigmoidoscope. In chronic diarrhoea, or diarrhoea associated with blood or mucus, a sigmoidoscopic examination is essential and should precede a barium enema.

Clinical assessment of dehydration in the elderly

Although dehydration is a frequent problem in the elderly, the criteria for the clinical assessment of this problem are meagre, in contrast to the extensive literature on assessment criteria in paediatric populations. Gross et al. (1992) conducted a prospective, correlational study with 55 subjects aged 60 or older, and concluded that the conventional signs and symptoms (derived from younger patients) are unreliable markers of dehydration in the elderly patient.

The conventional signs include: reduction of skin turgor, increased thirst, decreased peripheral perfusion, postural hypotension, low jugular venous pressure, patient sensations of thirst and dryness, tachycardia and high temperature. None of these symptoms or signs was shown to rank as a strong correlate of dehydration in the elderly. The reasons for the lack of correlation vary, but include the fact that there are normal age-related changes in these variables, and that the physiological responses to dehydration vary markedly between the elderly and younger patients. For example, postural hypotension is a common sign in the elderly patient, independent of the state of hydration due, possibly, to autonomic dysfunction and drug therapy.

Seven signs and symptoms are highlighted which strongly correlate with dehydration in the elderly, but are independent of significant, age-related change. They are:

- dry tongue
- longitudinal tongue furrows
- dry mucous membranes of nose and mouth
- eyes that appeared recessed in their sockets
- upper body muscle weakness
- speech difficulty
- confusion.

The time and effort spent in obtaining a comprehensive history and performing a complete physical examination will be rewarding for both patient and physician.

BIBLIOGRAPHY AND FURTHER READING

Gross, C.R., Lindquist, R.D., Woolley, A.C. et al. (1992). Clinical indicators of dehydration severity in elderly patients. *J. Emerg. Med.* **10**:267–74.

Holt, P.R. (1991). Approach to gastrointestinal problems in the elderly. In *Textbook of Gastroenterology,* vol 1, ed. T. Yamada, pp. 882–99. Philadelphia: Lippincott.

Matseshe, J.W. & Phillips, S.F. (1978). Chronic diarrhoea a practical approach. *Med. Clin. N. Am.* **62**:141–53.

Powell, D.W. (1991). Approach to the patient with diarrhoea. In *Textbook of Gastroenterology*, vol 1, ed. T. Yamada, pp. 732–78. Philadelphia: Lippincott.

Ratnaike, R.N. (1990). Diarrhoea in the elderly: epidemiological and aetiological factors. *J. Gastroenterol Hepatol* 5:449–58.

5 The investigation of diarrhoea

Joseph E. Buttery, Peter J. Lawson, Ranjit N. Ratnaike and
Anil B. Utturkar

The diagnosis of diarrhoea, due to the numerous causative factors, requires a multidisciplinary investigative approach. This chapter deals with several investigative procedures and laboratory tests.

The sections in this chapter are not prioritized to reflect greater importance to a particular specialty. For example, the decision whether to first request a stool microscopy and culture to identify an enteric pathogen or to request a double contrast barium study depends on the clinical circumstances.

INVASIVE PROCEDURES

Ranjit N. Ratnaike

Sigmoidoscopy is an extremely rewarding investigation and should be regarded as mandatory before a barium enema is performed. Sigmoidoscopy may reveal the presence of a tumour, lesions suggesting inflammatory bowel disease, ulceration due to infectious colitis, or plaques characteristic of pseudomembraneous colitis. In patients with proven bacillary dysentery, sigmoidoscopy is an extremely painful procedure and is unnecessary. A high rectal swab should be sent for immediate examination if a parasitic infection, for example amoebic dysentery, is suspected.

In diarrhoea suggesting large bowel pathology (diarrhoea with blood and mucus), the choice of the initial investigation lies between a double contrast barium enema (DCBE) and colonoscopy. In a study of 76 patients with colonic disease, colonoscopy was more accurate, particularly in the diagnosis of inflammatory bowel disease, where DCBE missed the diagnosis in 9 (64 per cent) of 14 patients. The advantages of colonoscopy include the opportunities to obtain biopsies and remove polyps.

HISTOLOGICAL INVESTIGATIONS

Ranjit N. Ratnaike

The small bowel biopsy

The major indication for a small bowel biopsy (SBB) is the suspicion of malabsorption. The small bowel biopsy is essential to diagnose small intestinal mucosal disease, as the main response to injury is alteration of villous architecture. In addition, the SBB provides a method to diagnose parasitic and fungal infection of the small intestine. Parasites which may be identified on small intestine biopsy are:

- *Giardia lamblia*
- *Cryptosporidium*
- *Microsporidia*
- *Isospora belli*
- *Sarcocystis hominis*
- *Strongyloides stercoralis.*

These parasitic infections do not cause distinctive histological features, but a specific diagnosis is possible by identifying the parasite in the mucosa.

Small bowel biopsies are now routinely obtained at endoscopy. These specimens, although smaller than those obtained with a biopsy capsule, usually pose no interpretive problems to pathologists. Endoscopy also allows for the convenient collection of intestinal juice for bacteriological culture and examination for parasitic pathogens.

In Western countries coeliac disease is the most common cause of villous atrophy. The entities listed below cause nonspecific small intestinal mucosal damage and the biopsy shows no distinctive features.

- coeliac disease
- severe bacterial infections
- giardiasis
- tropical sprue
- malnutrition
- dermatitis herpetiformis
- blind loop syndrome
- therapeutic agents: neomycin and colchicine.

In the diseases listed below the small bowel biopsy provides distinctive histological features to establish a diagnosis:

- Whipple's disease

- eosinophilic gastroenteritis
- lymphoma
- Crohn's disease
- adenocarcinoma
- Zollinger–Ellison syndrome
- amyloidosis.

Rectal biopsy

A rectal biopsy is indicated in patients with chronic diarrhoea of unknown aetiology and in whom there are sigmoidoscopic features of inflammation, or a tumour is present or amyloidosis is suspected. It is important that the rectal biopsy precedes a barium examination. The presence of barium complicates the interpretation of the histopathology of the specimen. As there is the potential for rectal perforation, especially in the elderly, the barium enema should be carried out at least a week after the biopsy.

HAEMATOLOGICAL INVESTIGATIONS

Ranjit N. Ratnaike

A haematological screen provides useful information to establish a diagnosis. In addition, haematological indices such as vitamin B_{12}, serum iron and folate reflect the severity and duration of malabsorption. Anaemia associated with diarrhoea may be due to iron, folate or, less commonly, vitamin B_{12} deficiency. The red cell morphology can vary from microcytosis in iron deficiency anaemia to macrocytosis from vitamin B_{12} deficiency.

A low haemoglobin and a low mean corpuscular volume (MCV) with erythrocyte morphology of iron deficiency, suggests the frequent occurrence of chronic occult blood loss and/or undernutrition in the elderly patient. A microcytic hypochromic anaemia may reflect malabsorption of iron due to a mucosal lesion of the upper small intestine. In coeliac disease, iron deficiency anaemia often dominates the clinical picture. Iron deficiency anaemia also occurs due to acute blood loss from inflammatory bowel disease, malignancy, severe dysentery and noninfective colitis. Chronic occult blood loss is a feature of inflammatory bowel disease. An early haematological abnormality of folate or vitamin B_{12} deficiency is an elevated MCV but may not occur if concurrent iron deficiency exists.

Howell–Jolly bodies are nuclear remnants in erythrocytes and are sometimes seen in the peripheral blood film of patients with coeliac disease with splenic atrophy. Hypersegmented neutrophils (neutrophils with six or seven lobes) are an early finding in vitamin B_{12} or folate deficiency and one particularly useful if the MCV is normal (e.g. if iron deficiency is also present). The following list shows the frequently encountered causes of eosinophilia, a useful diagnostic clue to the aetiology of diarrhoea.

Intestinal parasites

Protozoa

Isospora belli
Sarcocystis hominis.

Nematodes (round worms)

Strongyloides stercoralis
Trichuris trichura
Trichinella spiralis.

Trematodes (flukes)

Schistosoma mansoni
Schistosoma japonicum.

Other conditions

Eosinophilic gastroenteritis
Dermatitis herpetiformis
Inflammatory bowel disease.

An elevated eosinophil count is not an invariable manifestation of a parasitic infection. Eosinophilia occurs with *worm* infections, particularly helminths that invade tissue. A high eosinophil count as high as 20000 cells per µl of blood is seen with infections of *Strongyloides stercoralis*. The presence of eosinophilia as a side effect of therapeutic agents (erythromycin estolate, sulphonamides, chlorpropamide, p-aminosalicylic acid, imipramine, nitrofurantoin, procarbazine and methotrexate) for concurrent illness should also be considered.

A neutrophil leucocytosis and an elevated erythrocyte sedimentation rate (ESR) are frequent findings in inflammatory bowel disease, especially in Crohn's disease and, to a variable extent, in diarrhoea due to invasive bacterial pathogens.

The prothrombin time is prolonged in diseases of the small intestine due to vitamin K malabsorption. If a small intestinal biopsy is planned, treatment with vitamin K or an analogue is essential.

In patients with chronic diarrhoea the measurement of folate and vitamin B_{12}

levels are useful diagnostic pointers to small intestinal disease. Folate absorption occurs in the upper small intestine and vitamin B_{12} in the terminal ileum. Erythrocyte folate concentrations are a superior index of body stores as serum folate levels may rise soon after a folate-rich meal. In healthy adults the body stores of folate last up to three months. In the elderly the folate stores may be drastically depleted due to undernutrition, or to treatment with drugs such as phenytoin or barbiturates, or to excessive alcohol intake.

Low folate concentrations are usually seen with chronic mucosal injury to the upper small intestine that occurs in coeliac disease, tropical sprue or as a result of treatment with drugs such as neomycin, colchicine and methotrexate. Other causes of folate deficiency associated with diarrhoea include bacterial overgrowth of the small intestine (see Chapter 9) and Crohn's disease (see Chapter 12). Despite upper small intestinal damage, an acute episode of diarrhoea, for example with rotavirus, does not decrease folate levels.

A normal vitamin B_{12} concentration does not exclude malabsorption since body stores of vitamin B_{12} last for 3–5 years. Decreased vitamin B_{12} concentrations suggest long standing disease and possible causes are:

- bacterial overgrowth
- Crohn's disease
- coeliac disease
- tropical sprue
- ulcerative colitis
- ileal resection
- ileal bypass involving the terminal ileum.

It is important that low vitamin B_{12} levels be further investigated by the Schilling test. The test, carried out with and without intrinsic factor, will exclude pernicious anaemia as a cause of vitamin B_{12} deficiency. In states of bacterial overgrowth bacteria compete with the host for luminal vitamin B_{12} and consume more than the host absorbs.

MICROBIOLOGICAL INVESTIGATIONS

Peter J. Lawson

The specimen

Ideally, a fresh sample of 20 to 40 g of stool should be examined within 30 minutes of collection. While some organisms responsible for diarrhoea are quite hardy, others succumb to the fall in pH, drying, and the accumulation of products of bacterial metabolism. Similarly, leucocytes and amoebic trophozoites are rapidly disrupted after passage of the stool.

Microbiologists are often amused to receive a request form with diarrhoea as the reason for sending a pellet of faeces so hard that it rattles when the container is shaken. It is important that the specimen submitted is consistent with clinical expectations before accepting a negative microscopy and culture result.

Most laboratories will provide, as part of their report, a macroscopic description of the specimen. The stool appearance, along with presence of pus and blood, is a guide whether the diarrhoea, if bacterial, is of a penetrating inflammatory type, as in Shigellosis, or the watery toxin-mediated type like cholera.

Microbiology laboratories tend to 'tailor' their examination of a stool specimen subject to the macroscopic appearance, clinical information provided and local knowledge such as the requesting specialty and current epidemiology. For example, a history of recent seafood ingestion is a valuable pointer to inoculate *Vibrio* isolation media. A history of immune deficiency warrants a workup that includes examination for *Cryptosporidium* and other parasites.

Basic laboratory procedures

Pathogens detectable on microscopy

In the laboratory, areas of the stool that appear mucoid or bloody are emulsified into a drop of saline on a slide and examined for white and red blood cells and parasites. Stains such as methylene blue, phloxine, iodine or eosin, are used to identify cells, trophozoites and cysts.

A rigorous examination for parasites includes a stool concentration method using salt or sugar flotation, or more often a formol–ether centrifugation process. Trophozoite and cyst identification is based on size and fine structure using high-power microscopy on fixed smears stained with an iron-haematoxylin stain.

The presence of many leucocytes in the stool suggests large intestinal pathology of inflammatory origin. Leucocytes are detected in the faeces by microscopy on a wet preparation stained with Loeffler's methylene blue.

Some microscopic features used to identify protozoa are as follows.

Parasites

Giardia lamblia

Motile *Giardia* are detected in a saline wet mount of a liquid stool or duodenal aspirate by their vigorous activity, and identified by the overall leaf-like shape and distinctive internal features. In formed stools, the cysts can be concentrated by the formol–ether or flotation techniques, and are identifiable by their axostyle and other internal features.

Entamoeba histolytica

E. histolytica may be detected in warm saline mounts of fresh liquid stool. A positive identification is based on the presence of ingested red blood cells and on size and nuclear and cytoplasmic detail best seen with iron-haematoxylin staining.

Blastocystis hominis

This protozoan has been associated with diarrhoea. It is generally seen in saline wet stool mounts in a vacuolated form, 8–10 μm in diameter, often with a prominent slime capsule.

Cryptosporidium species

This organism is detected by making a smear of the specimen on a slide, which is then heat fixed and stained with a modified Kinyoun acid-fast stain similar to that used for *Mycobacterium tuberculosis*. The parasites are stained with sufficient contrast so that they are relatively easily recognized against the background of faecal bacteria and debris.

Isospora belli and *Sacrocystis hominis*

Isospora belli is best detected and identified in modified acid-fast (Kinyoun) stained preparations. The oocyst is an elliptical acid-fast structure 22 to 33 by 10 to 15 μm, often showing two internal sporocysts. *S. hominis* is similar in appearance, but the oocyst is more regularly ovoid in shape.

Balantidium coli

This large ciliate protozoan is a relatively uncommon parasite of humans. It is easily identified in saline wet mounts from its size (50–200 μm) and peripheral cilia.

Bacteria

Most laboratories choose their basic media to recover *Salmonella*, *Shigella* and *Campylobacter*. In the hospital setting particularly, an attempt will be made to check for *Clostridium difficile* by culture, toxin detection, or both. Less common pathogens such as *Aeromonas*, *Yersinia* and *Vibrio* can be detected by experienced microbiologists on the basic *Salmonella–Shigella* media set, although more specific media yield a better chance of isolation.

It is the minor differences in nutritional activity and resistance to toxic compounds of these organisms that are exploited in the complex culture media used to isolate them.

The wide choice of differential–selective agar media currently popular in laboratories for the isolation of *Salmonella* sp. and *Shigella* sp. are xylose–lysine–desoxy-cholate (XLD), *Salmonella–Shigella* (SS) and MacConkey medium. A laboratory will commonly use two of these to increase isolation rates. The media contain a variety of compounds, such as bile salts, that selectively suppress growth of some normal bowel flora, for example *Escherichia* and *Enterococcus*, while allowing a minority population of *Salmonella* or *Shigella* to grow.

The media are also rendered 'differential' by including a nutrient substrate, such as lactose, along with a pH indicator. Organisms that ferment lactose produce lactic acid, resulting in a red-coloured colony. More complex and elegant biochemical differentiators of nutritional activity can be used, such as are present in XLD medium to show the decarboxylation of xylose and lysine.

One or more types of enrichment broth will be inoculated. For example, selenite broth and Rappaport's medium are formulated to support preferentially the growth of some pathogenic species of interest while suppressing or holding static the numbers of the normal bowel flora.

The agar plates are streaked and incubated for 18 to 24 hours.

After incubation, plates are examined for 'suspect' colonies. Growth from a faecal inoculum on selective–differential media is rarely pure, even in the case of a florid Salmonellosis and colonies are not easily distinguishable from Proteus by their pale colour on a medium containing lactose since both organisms are non-lactose fermenters. Therefore, several of each morphological type of suspect colony are 'picked off' and subcultured into a range of differential broth media. Proteus, for instance, are rapidly screened out by their ability to split urea to ammonia.

Various commercially prepared differential sugar identification systems for enterobacteriaceae are now employed widely. These consist of plastic strips or plates containing moulded wells or bubbles, into which sugar or substrate mixtures, along with indicator agents, have been freeze-dried.

A suspension of a suspect organism is added to each well, rehydrating the material as it is inoculated. After incubation, results are interpreted by noting the colour change in each well. The results can be recorded as a number by assigning positive and negative results in a binary fashion, as ones and zeros. Sequential groups are then added together to produce a 'biogram' signature that reflects the activity of the organism in a wide range of substrates. The companies marketing these systems supply lists of numbers that correlate a specific biogram with ranked identity probabilities, determined from large databases of reference organisms. Several automated systems (e.g. Vitek) are available that handle all the steps from inoculation through to identification with a combination of mechanical, optical and computer technologies.

Bacterial agents detectable in culture

Staphylococcus aureus

Laboratory confirmation involves demonstration of the organism in food or faeces, or the detection of one of the five heat-resistant staphylococcal enterotoxins in gel diffusion or radioimmunoassay (RIA) tests.

Bacillus cereus and Clostridium perfringens

Both organisms cause food poisoning. Laboratory confirmation depends on the demonstration of high counts of bacteria in the faeces of affected individuals and in the ingested food.

Clostridium difficile

This organism can be isolated from faeces by use of antibiotic-containing selective media, and identified by carbohydrate fermentation and gas–liquid chromatography of its metabolic products. Toxin detection methods include a cell-culture cytotoxicity technique on faecal extracts, and the detection of an associated protein by a commercial latex particle agglutination on a faecal suspension.

Enterotoxigenic, invasive, adherent and haemorrhagic E. coli

E. coli is normally present in stool cultures in large numbers. Pathogenic strains are classified on their harbouring of plasmids or phages that encode for a variety of pathogenic mechanisms.

Although certain sero groups have been associated with each of these classes of E. coli, the transmissible plasmid or phage-borne nature of their pathogenicity makes sero group detection unreliable. The detection of these organisms in the clinical laboratory awaits the development of new techniques in molecular biology.

Salmonella

Many selective media have been produced that use the resistance of Salmonella to a range of compounds, including bile salts, selenium salts and dyes. The organisms are classically motile, nonlactose fermenters, oxidase and urease negative. Isolates of Salmonella are generally reported generically by laboratories as 'Salmonella species'. A follow-up report is issued when the isolate is further identified to one of the thousand or so known species. This extra species information may be useful in tracing a source of infection.

Where a fever is present in patients with Salmonella, the organism can frequently be isolated from blood cultures.

Shigella species

Molecular biology has revealed that the four *Shigella* species and *E. coli* are so closely related as to be the same species based on DNA hybridization. *Shigella* species are isolated readily on the less selective enteric media such as XLD, and identified by carbohydrate reactions. Shigellae are nonmotile, and are usually lactose nonfermenters.

Yersinia enterocolitica

A specialized selective media (CIN agar) is available for the isolation of *Y. enterocolitica*. The organism is somewhat peculiar in that it grows better at lower temperatures (22 to 25°C) than other *Enterobacteraceae*. This characteristic is used to enhance isolation of pathogen by storing a saline emulsion of the stool at 4°C for one to three weeks and subculturing onto MacConkey agar at room temperature. Laboratories more commonly store a MacConkey agar plate at room temperature for two to four days and examine it for suspect colonies that have enlarged appreciably at the lower temperature on the bench. The organism is a motile lactose and oxidase negative urease producer that does not deaminate phenylalanine. Test results differ markedly at 22 to 37°C, motility and various other reactions being negative at the higher temperature.

Aeromonas hydrophila

This organism can be isolated from faeces using media that select for its usual resistance to ampicillin, but this characteristic is not invariable. *Aeromonas* is motile, oxidase positive and variably ferments lactose.

Vibrio cholerae and Vibrio parahaemolyticus

The reliable isolation of *Vibrio* species requires the use of specialized media such as TCBS. The two species are oxidase positive, but differ in that *V. parahaemolyticus* is halophilic, i.e. it has a requirement for sodium chloride. Both organisms are readily identified by carbohydrate fermentation.

Campylobacter

This microaerophilic, thermophilic organism requires an isolation medium that contains antibiotics as selective agents and supplements of blood or charcoal to overcome the toxic effects of peroxides that occur in organic substrates exposed to air. Isolation media are incubated at 43°C in an atmosphere of 3–5 per cent oxygen in carbon dioxide or nitrogen for 48 to 72 hours. Isolates are identified by their curved shape in gram-stain, darting motility in wet preparation microscopy and positive oxidase reaction. Pus and blood are not uncommon in the stools of infected patients, and the organism may appear in blood cultures from some patients.

Viral agents

Rotavirus

Enzyme-linked immunosorbent assay (ELISA) tests are the diagnostic tests routinely used. The virus can be cultured with difficulty.

Norwalk-like agents

Immune electron-microscopy may be used to detect the infectious particle, but is usually regarded only as a research technique. Various RIA and ELISA methods under development may prove useful in the future.

BIOCHEMICAL INVESTIGATIONS

Joseph E. Buttery

Biochemical tests which are useful in the diagnosis and management of diarrhoea are discussed in this section.

Blood

The loss of bicarbonate in diarrhoea leads to low plasma bicarbonate concentration. This then lowers the blood pH (Henderson–Hasselbalch equation) causing metabolic acidosis. The acid–base status should be monitored when the plasma bicarbonate is very low by measuring blood pH and arterial blood gases. If acidosis is severe, bicarbonate therapy may be required.

Potassium loss in the diarrhoeal fluid leads to hypokalaemia. If the patient is also hypovolaemic, more potassium is lost in the urine due to secondary hyperaldosteronism. Most patients with severe diarrhoea will present with hypokalaemic hyperchloraemic metabolic acidosis.

Hypomagnesaemia can occur with prolonged diarrhoea and its measurement may be warranted on clinical grounds or as a routine investigation. Endocrine disorders that cause diarrhoea and the tests to diagnose these conditions are listed in Table 5.1. Most of these tests are not routinely measured in hospital laboratories and are usually sent away to specialized centres.

Diarrhoea causes the loss of water, sodium, potassium and bicarbonate. Direct water loss cannot easily be measured by most laboratories, and indirect tests to measure the resulting hypovolaemia are: plasma specific gravity, plasma proteins (albumin and globulins), osmolality, urea, and creatinine.

Severe hypovolaemia will cause the concentrations of all these test results to be raised. Recently, the measurement of plasma specific gravity was re-evaluated to identify hypovolaemia, especially in the older adults. The test relies on determin-

Table 5.1. Biochemical tests used to investigate patients with endocrine disorders

Disease	Test
Zollinger–Ellison syndrome (gastrinoma)	Plasma gastrin
Verner–Morrison syndrome (VIPoma)	Plasma vasoactive intestinal peptide
Glucagonoma	Plasma glucagon
Carcinoid syndrome	Plasma serotonin
Somatostatinoma	Plasma somatostatin
Hyperthyroidism	Plasma T_4, TSH
Medullary thyroid carcinoma	Plasma calcitonin, CEA

ing the plasma refractive index with a hand-held refractometer; the specific gravity is determined using a standard conversion table. The test can be rapidly performed and is reported to be accurate. However, falsely elevated (e.g. hypergammaglobulin-aemia, multiple myeloma) and increased values are obtained in certain clinical conditions since the refractive index of any fluid is a direct measure of the total mass of large molecules in solution.

Hypovolaemia increases the renal absorption of sodium and chloride, which tends to normalize the plasma sodium and increase the plasma chloride concentrations. If this dehydration is corrected with only water (nonisotonic), hyponatraemia can occur with normal plasma chloride concentration.

Urine

In cases of diarrhoea with suspected laxative abuse, the analysis of urine is preferred to blood or faeces as the urine test is the most sensitive. In the investigation of diarrhoea of unknown origin an early screen for urine laxatives is particularly useful among the elderly as a cost-effective procedure. The screening should detect the presence of the diphenolic laxatives that include phenolphthalein and bisacodyl, and the anthraquinones that include senna and danthron. The testing of a second urine sample is recommended to confirm the suspicion of laxative abuse.

Elevated urinary excretion of 5-hydroxyindole acetic acid from a 24-hour urine sample is a test to diagnose the carcinoid syndrome. The diarrhoea which is explosive and watery is a prominent feature in about 5 per cent of patients who show any symptoms.

Blood and urine

The oral 5 or 25 g xylose absorption test is sometimes used to assess intestinal malabsorption. A low plasma and urine xylose concentration suggests intestinal malabsorption. The reliability of this test, especially in the elderly, is dubious as most have mild renal impairment that affects xylose excretion. Also, bacterial overgrowth metabolizes unabsorbed xylose and can cause spuriously low xylose excretion.

Faeces

The measurement of faecal fluid osmolality and electrolytes may be used to determine the nature of the diarrhoea. Faecal osmolality is a measure of faecal water osmolality. The faeces are centrifuged and the supernatant assayed for osmolality, sodium and potassium. The osmolality thus obtained is the *measured* osmolality. The *calculated* osmolality is determined from the concentrations of Na and K, as $(Na + K) \times 2$.

Osmotic gap = *measured* osmolality − *calculated* osmolality

The osmotic gap shows whether the diarrhoea is secretory or osmotic.

In secretory diarrhoea there is abnormal secretion of fluid and electrolytes into the intestine. The diarrhoea is usually large volume (> 1.0 l/day) and persists even when the patient has fasted. The *measured* and *calculated* osmolalities are usually the same and the osmotic gap is either low or absent.

Osmotic diarrhoea, on the other hand, is caused by the presence of unabsorbed osmotically active substances in the intestine. These compounds are usually carbohydrates, saline laxatives, $MgSO_4$ or various sodium salts. The volume of diarrhoea can be large but is considerably reduced when the patient has fasted. The *measured* osmolality is much higher, due to the presence of solutes, than the *calculated* osmolality and, consequently, the osmotic gap is high, usually 50 to 100 mmol/kg or even much higher. Magnesium-based laxatives or antacids will cause the *measured* osmolality to be elevated but not the *calculated* osmolality (as this measures only the Na and K). Hence, the osmotic gap is large.

Sulphate or phosphate ingestion should be suspected when the faecal Na, K and osmolality are all excessively raised. The presence of SO_4 in faecal water can be tested by the addition of barium chloride solution that forms a white precipitate of barium sulphate. Osmotic diarrhoea due to carbohydrate malabsorption usually causes low stool pH of about 5 (normal about pH 7) while osmotic diarrhoea due to poorly absorbed salts causes stool pH to be around 7–8. A faecal Mg concentration greater than 12 mmol/l strongly suggests the ingestion of a magnesium-containing drug.

There is still controversy regarding the ideal faecal collection for measuring the osmotic gap. A 24-hour collection is widely used, but a three-day collection from a patient fasted and maintained on fluid infusion has been recommended. It is difficult to differentiate between secretory and osmotic diarrhoea based on the osmotic gap when the faecal volume is less than 500 ml/day. The storage of faeces at room temperature of 25 °C for 24 hours has been shown to increase faecal fluid osmolality and, hence, the osmotic gap. This observation can have serious implications on the usefulness of measuring the osmotic gap. Confusion may arise if the stool is tampered with water (faecal osmolality less than plasma osmolality) or with urine (faecal osmolality is greater than plasma osmolality).

The measurement of faecal Mg, SO_4 and PO_4 can sometimes be useful in detecting the surreptitious use of laxatives.

Chronic diarrhoea could be due to fat malabsorption. If so, the faecal fat concentration is raised (steatorrhoea). The fat in faeces is derived from the unabsorbed dietary fat and this could be due to either an intestinal or a pancreatic disease. For a reliable faecal fat test a three-day stool collection is required. Ideally the patient should be maintained on a 100 g fat per day diet for three days before the three-day collection. This protocol is more difficult to follow in elderly patients and therefore the simple qualitative test for excess fat in the stool still has a role and can suggest a diagnosis of modest or severe steatorrhoea.

The detection of laxatives in faeces is sometimes carried out but is of limited use. Phenolphthalein laxative can easily be detected by the addition of alkali to the faecal water sample where a pink colour forms. Use of urine samples is preferred for the investigation of laxative abuse.

Breath tests

The investigation of diarrhoea in the elderly suspected of lactose intolerance or bacterial overgrowth should preferably be noninvasive and convenient for the patient.

Breath testing procedures to diagnose deficiency of the lactase enzyme and bacterial overgrowth in the small intestine do not involve intubation. On the other hand, the tests are often lengthy and inconvenient. Two breath tests are used frequently: the lactose H_2 breath test is used to diagnose lactose intolerance due to lactase deficiency, and the ^{14}C-xylose breath test is used to diagnose bacterial overgrowth of the small intestine.

The lactose breath test is performed by administering an oral 50 g lactose solution and measuring the expired breath H_2. In the absence of lactase, the unabsorbed lactose is metabolized by the enteric bacteria to produce H_2. A breath H_2 concentration greater than 20 ppm over the basal value indicates lactase deficiency and, hence, lactose intolerance. Unfortunately, there are problems associated with this test, one of which is the absence of H_2-producing bacteria in about 5 to 15 per cent of the population. A new ^{13}C lactose probe which measures the $^{13}CO_2$ in the patient's breath, and hence directly assesses lactose absorption, is likely to supersede the breath H_2 test.

The ^{14}C-xylose breath test is performed by ingesting 1 g of xylose containing about 10 µCi of ^{14}C-xylose, and measuring the breath radioactive CO_2 concentration after 30 and 60 minutes. If elevated, this confirms the presence of bacterial overgrowth in the small intestine. A variation of this test is to use nonradioactive xylose. This involves the administration of 25 g of xylose and the measurement of H_2 in the expired breath samples. A raised H_2 concentration in the breath sample indicates bacterial overgrowth. This test has yet to be fully validated.

The ^{14}C-triolein breath test for fat malabsorption, which measures $^{14}CO_2$ excretion in the breath, is showing promise as a diagnostically useful test. Erroneous results may occur in patients with other diseases such as diabetes mellitus, thyroid disorders, hyperlipidaemia, chronic liver disease, and lung disease.

In severe diarrhoea, blood pH and electrolyte measurements will ascertain the extent of electrolyte loss, so that immediate treatment can be started to replace these losses via intravenous fluid and electrolyte therapy. The analysis of urine may produce information regarding the surreptitious use of laxatives. Faecal electrolyte and osmolality may explain the nature of the diarrhoea. Specific hormone tests in blood may confirm endocrine disorders causing the diarrhoea.

RADIOLOGICAL INVESTIGATIONS

Anil B. Utturkar

When a patient presents with diarrhoea intrinsic abnormalities of the small or large intestine as the primary pathology are considered. It is important, however, to remember the extrinsic causes of diarrhoea, such as metabolic disorders, endocrine causes, pancreatic abnormalities, drugs and the irritable bowel syndrome. Spurious diarrhoea can occur secondary to faecal incontinence. Previous gastrointestinal surgery is another important cause.

The radiological investigations consist of plain x-rays of the abdomen, barium enema and follow-through examinations. Depending on the clinical indications, CT scanning, ultrasound examination and cholangiography may be required. A chest x-ray also may be necessary.

Plain x-rays

If the diarrhoea is due to infective, metabolic, endocrine or small intestinal causes, the plain x-rays of the abdomen are not rewarding. Often in the erect view slight distension of the small and/or large bowel loops with a few fluid levels are seen. In cancer of the colon, plain x-rays may show intestinal obstruction in the form of

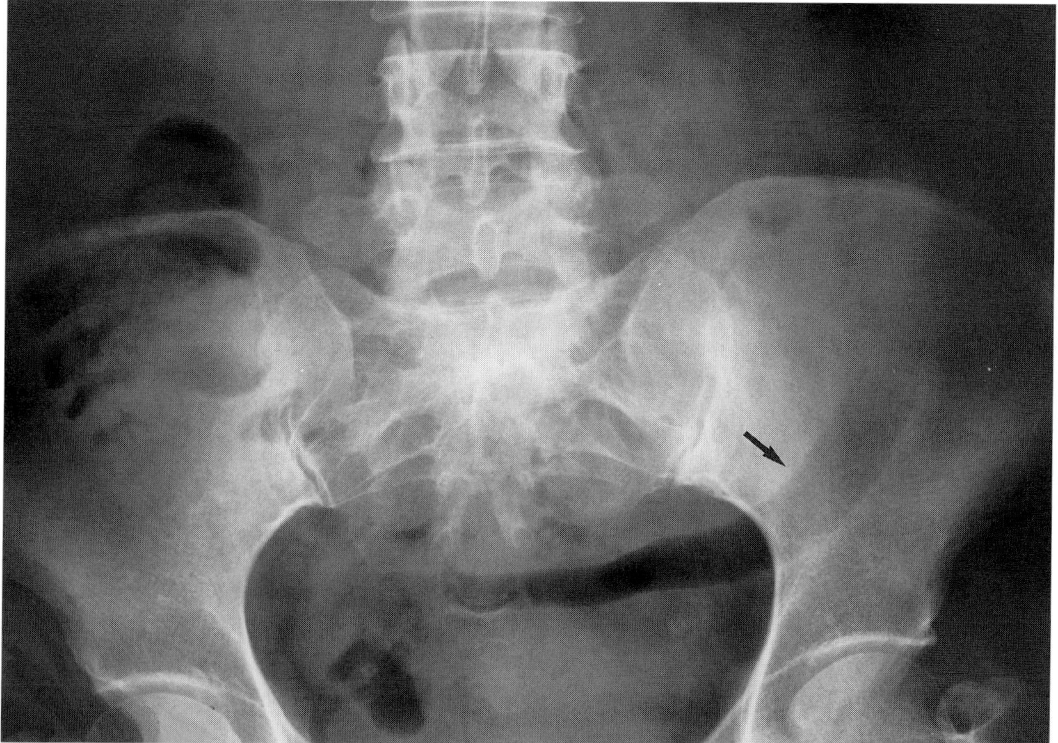

Figure 5.1.　Featureless lower descending and sigmoid colon showing 'hose pipe' appearance and shortening in chronic ulcerative colitis.

gross gaseous distension of the bowel loops, with multiple fluid levels arranged in step-ladder pattern.

In cases of inflammatory bowel disease there may be evidence of a localized segment of toxic megacolon (acute toxic dilatation of the colon). The transverse colon is affected most often and the colonic diameter is usually more than 6 cm. The normal haustral pattern is lost and there is thickening of the bowel wall with mucosal excrescences giving an irregular outline to the gas-filled colon. The affected portion of the colon is paralysed producing 'functional obstruction'. A toxic megacolon usually implies possible rupture. These changes are usually nonspecific and similar appearances are seen in cases of ischaemic and pseudo-membraneous colitis. Often, an affected segment of the colon is seen as a tubular, adynamic segment with loss of haustration and some mucosal oedema. This usually implies chronic changes (Figure 5.1).

Faecal loading with slight distension of the colonic loops is evident in cases of spurious diarrhoea and faecal incontinence. In colonic pseudo-obstruction, there is even more distension of the large bowel loops with some fluid levels. These

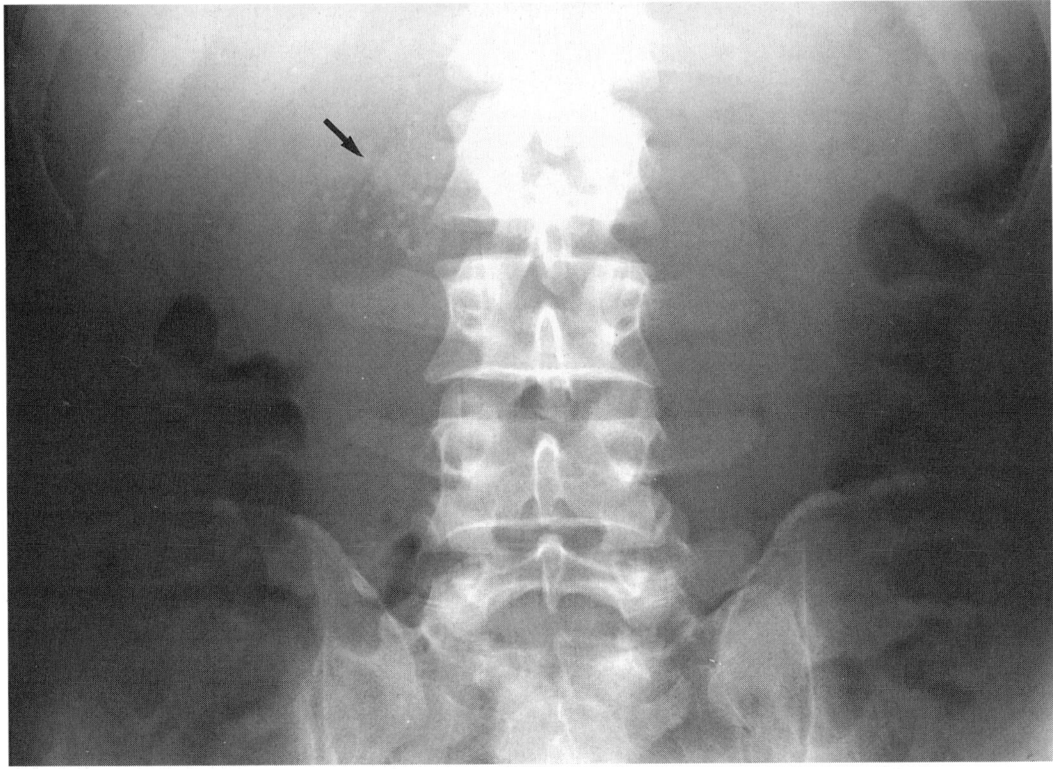

Figure 5.2.   Calcification in the pancreas in chronic pancreatitis.

patients usually tend to be fairly elderly, often immobile with illness or injury and are also on treatment involving antiparkinsonian, antidepressant drugs and pheno-thiazines.

If the diarrhoea is due to pancreatic causes, calcification may be visible along the long axis of the pancreas (Figure 5.2). Fine sand-like calcification in the liver may give a clue to an underlying mucus-secreting malignancy of the bowel. Very rarely calcification may occur in a primary tumour.

Barium enema

Inflammatory bowel disease, diverticular disease and ischaemic and neoplastic lesions of the colon are among the common causes of diarrhoea in the elderly. A barium enema is an important investigation.

The colonic cancers are seen as polypoidal filling defects or narrowed segments or strictures. The latter usually have 'shoulders' and produce the classically described 'apple-core' appearance (Figure 5.3). A plaque-like cancer is evident only

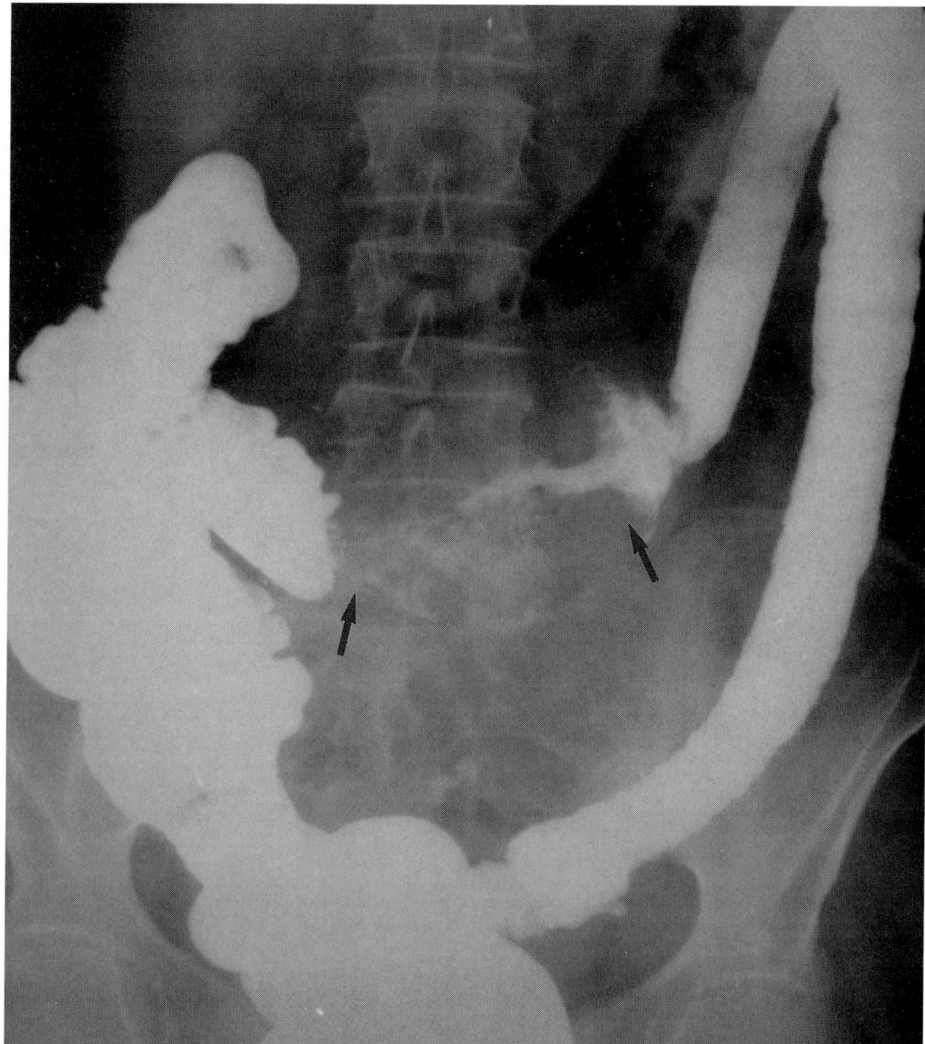

Figure 5.3.   Carcinoma of the colon. An 'apple core' lesion in the transverse colon.

occasionally. In villous adenomas, a large polypoidal mass with multiple fronds is seen commonly in the rectum and caecum, but can occur elsewhere.

In cases of diverticular disease, there are multiple flask-like outpouchings from the bowel wall and the necks of the diverticula are usually narrow. Often there is associated bowel spasm that results in local contraction, producing a 'saw-tooth' appearance (Figure 5.4). The affected segment of the colon is usually shortened and thickened, and tender on palpation. There is occasionally evidence of complicating features such as perforation, resulting in pneumoperitoneum. Pericolic abscess may be evident as an extrinsic impression with narrowing of the lumen that tends to be

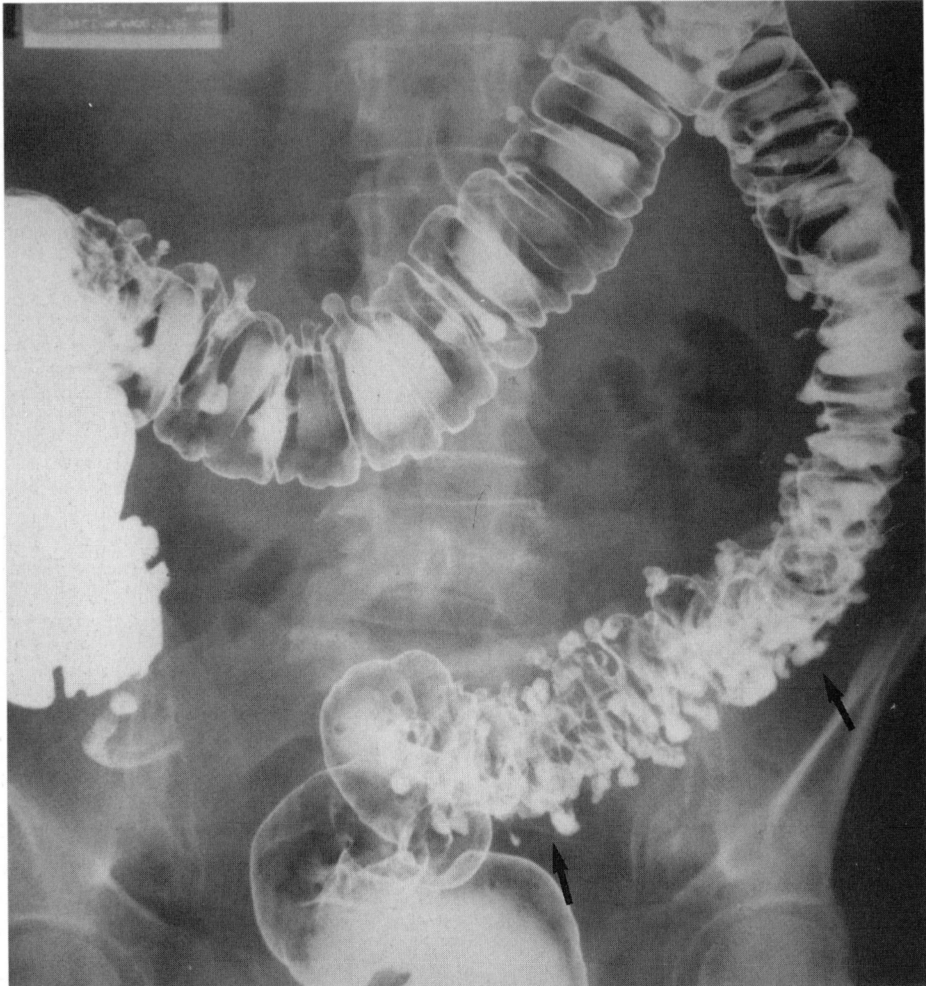

Figure 5.4.   Diverticular disease. Multiple flask-like outpouchings of the colon. Note hypertrophy of the circular muscle folds and accentuation of the haustral pattern.

eccentric. Sinuses or fistulas are common and, when they occur, usually communicate with the colon or urinary bladder and vagina and, very rarely, with the skin.

In the irritable bowel syndrome there is usually bowel spasm and very rapid transit of the barium, with functional narrowing of the lumen and a 'saw-tooth' appearance very similar to that seen in cases of diverticular disease; but diverticula are absent. The spasm is usually relieved after intravenous injection of buscopan or glucagon, and the colon can distend reasonably well depending upon severity of the bowel spasm. In ischaemic colitis, there is 'thumb-printing' of the colonic mucosa due to submucosal bleeding (Figure 5.5). These changes, however, are often tran-

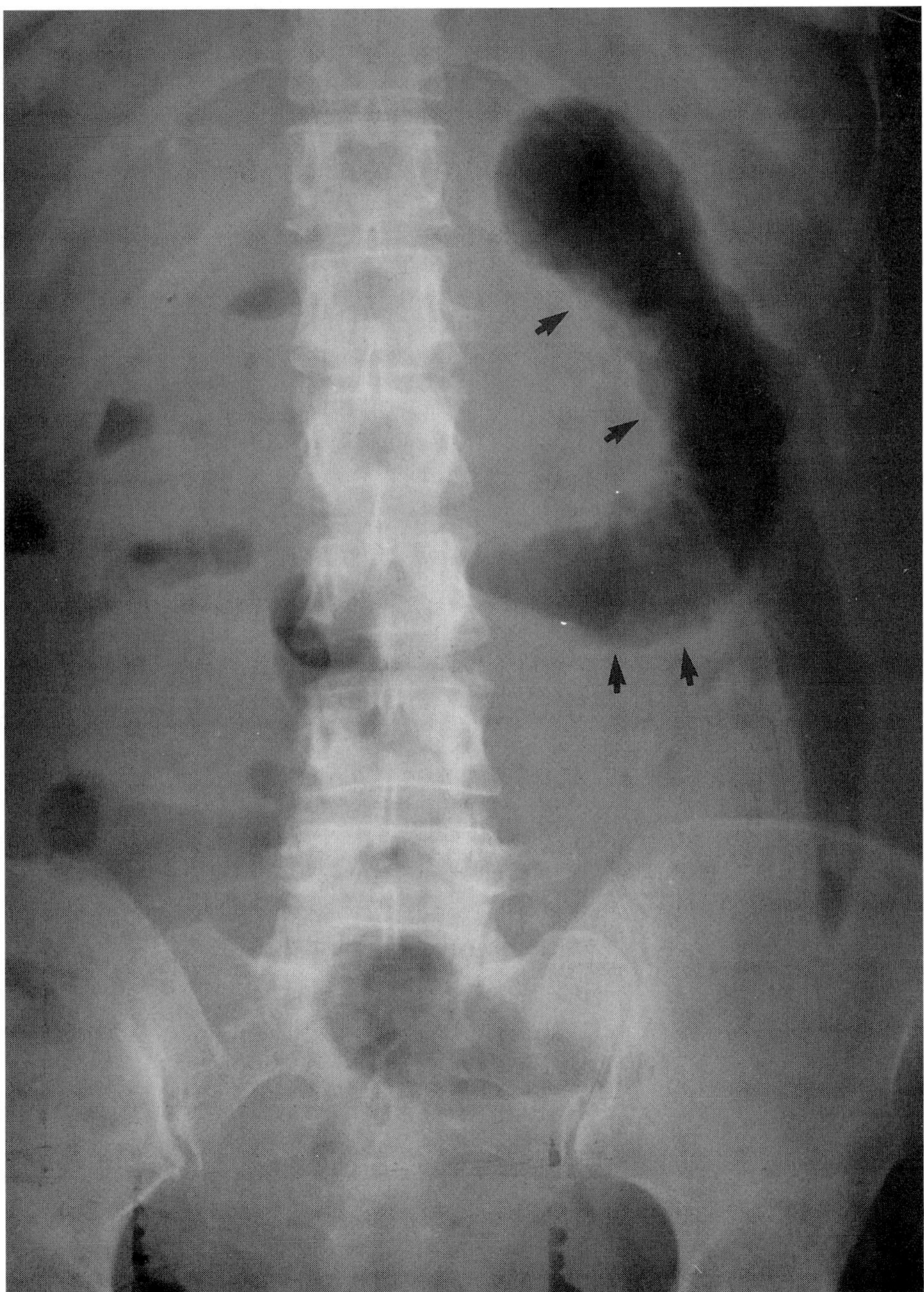

Figure 5.5.   'Thumb printing' in ischaemic colitis.

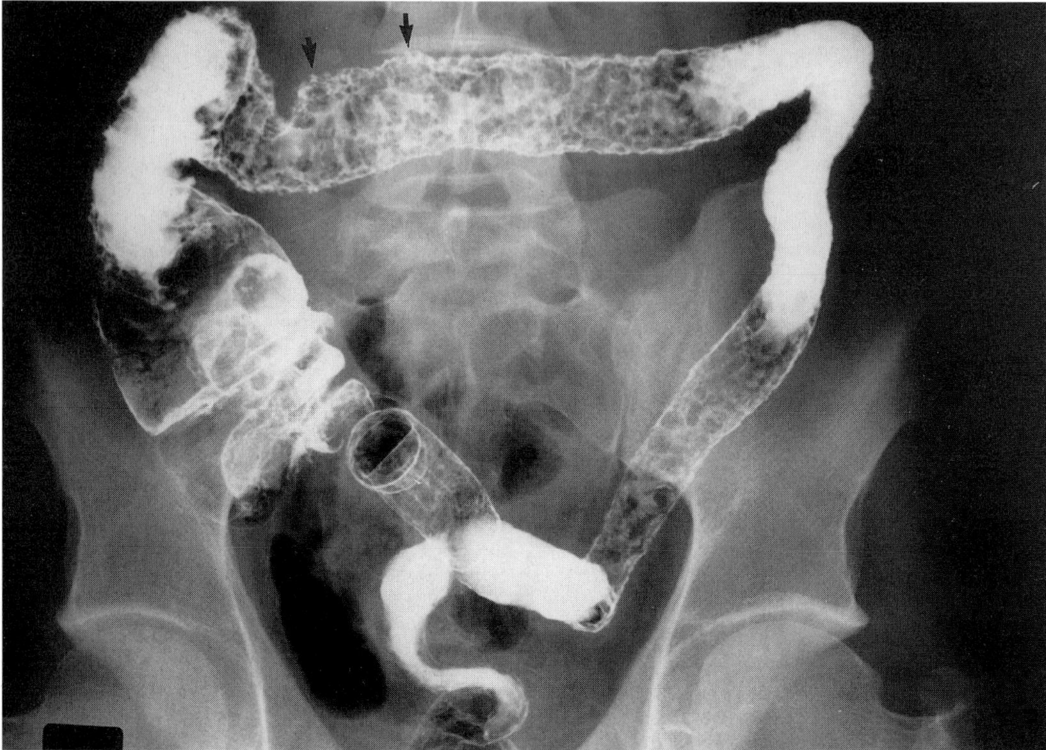

Figure 5.6.   Ulcerative colitis. Fine ulceration, 'collar-stud' ulcers, discontinuous mucosal line and coarse granular appearance.

sient and can be effaced with colonic distension, and are better seen on single contrast enema. In advanced cases one may see a pseudotumour caused by thickening of the bowel wall and intramural haemorrhage. The pseudotumour usually disappears if collateral circulation is adequate.

Inflammatory bowel diseases produce characteristic changes on barium enema. An overlap in the radiological findings occurs in Crohn's disease and ulcerative colitis. In ulcerative colitis, the involvement of the colon is retrograde from rectum upwards and is usually continuous. Early changes show loss of definition of the sharp mucosal line and there is fine granularity. As the disease progresses, the granular appearance becomes coarse and the mucosal line, when seen in profile, appears discontinuous and somewhat beaded. Frank ulceration is evident but the ulcers tend to be shallow. The larger ulcers assume a classical 'collar-stud' appearance and can coalesce (Figures. 5.6 and 5.7). There is often polypoidal appearance due to inflammatory changes. As the disease advances the colon shortens and the lumen narrows with loss of haustration, and subsequent effacement occurs. In initial stages the effacement is due to oedema of the mucosa and submucosa, resulting in

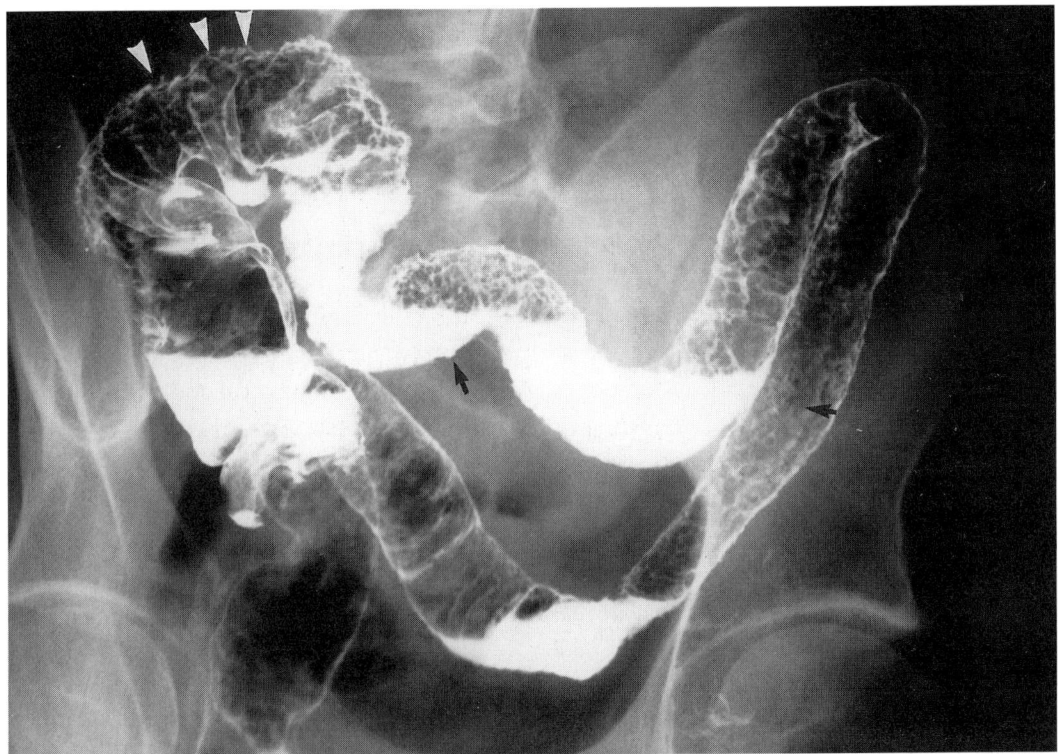

Figure 5.7.   Ulcerative colitis. Fine ulceration, 'collar-stud' ulcers, discontinuous mucosal line and coarse granular appearance.

thickening and blunting of mucosal folds with smoothing out of primary folds and valvulae conniventes. Subsequently, there is involvement of the muscularis layer. In chronic stages 'hose pipe' deformity is evident. Perforation can occur if there is toxic megacolon which is a serious complication. Linear streaks of gas in the colonic wall are seen and indicate potential necrosis and impending rupture of the bowel wall.

Malignant change is not uncommon and is directly proportional to the chronicity of the disease. There is a 20 per cent chance of cancer developing in a patient with a 20-year history of ulcerative colitis. The cancer is usually plaque-like or scirrhous and causes a stricture, and differentiation from a benign stricture can be exceedingly difficult.

In Crohn's disease the inflammation is transmural rather than submucosal, and the inflammatory changes involve the entire thickness of the bowel wall. Characteristically, the mucosal line is discontinuous along the length and circumferentially. The mucosal involvement is patchy and the earliest feature is the 'aphthoid' ulcer producing 'bulls-eye' or 'target' lesions. The ulcers tend to be deep and are occasionally thorn-shaped (pointed). The ulceration can be deep and linear and a combination of these, with mucosal oedema, produces the 'cobblestone' appearance. The haustral loss is often irregular and eccentric, and produces the classical 'purse-string' appearance (Figure 5.8). Skip lesions with intervening areas of normal mucosa are characteristic and strictures are common. Internal fistulas with other organs and fistulous communications with the skin are also features of this disease. Involvement of the terminal ileum is quite characteristic (Figure 5.9). In 50 per cent of the cases, the rectum is spared. Despite the many characteristic features, differentiation from other lesions is quite difficult. For example, aphthoid ulcers are also seen in *Yersinia* enterocolitis while involvement of the ileocaecal region is seen in cases of tuberculosis, amoebiasis and *Yersinia* infections. Pseudomembraneous colitis is also difficult to distinguish from inflammatory bowel disease, as the radiological features overlap and consist predominantly of an alteration of the mucosal pattern with mucosal oedema, loss of haustration and a diffusely irregular, shaggy appearance of bowel wall resembling ulceration. Amoebiasis involves the colon, especially the ascending colon, and the ileocaecal region. Sometimes a localized granulomatous lesion may develop, producing a mass in the caecum (amoeboma) which mimics cancer.

Barium meal and follow-through

The malabsorption syndrome is a common cause of chronic diarrhoea. This can be broadly divided into two groups.

Group I shows radiological features of steatorrhoea that include diseases with diffuse lesions of intestinal mucosa, such as coeliac disease, tropical sprue, Whipple's disease and amyloidosis. A subgroup in this category includes diseases that cause steatorrhoea due to maldigestion: a deficiency of pancreatic juice in chronic pancreatitis or a lack of bile salts in obstructive jaundice or primary biliary cirrhosis. In all these conditions the radiological findings are nonspecific.

The radiological features consist of dilatation of the small intestinal loops and there is often segmentation and flocculation and clumping of the barium. The calibre of the small bowel is directly proportional to the extent of the disease (Figures. 5.10 and 5.11). In Whipple's disease the changes are similar but nonspecific. Enlarged lymph nodes are present and there is sclerosis of the sacroiliac joints that suggests the diagnosis. The bone changes in the spine resemble rheumatoid arthritis. The final diagnosis should be established by intestinal biopsy.

The group II diseases of malabsorption usually show *specific* radiological features consisting of localized lesions of the small intestine such as in Crohn's disease, lymphoma and scleroderma. In Crohn's disease the small bowel changes are similar to those seen in the colon, and consist of ulceration, mucosal thickening, matting of

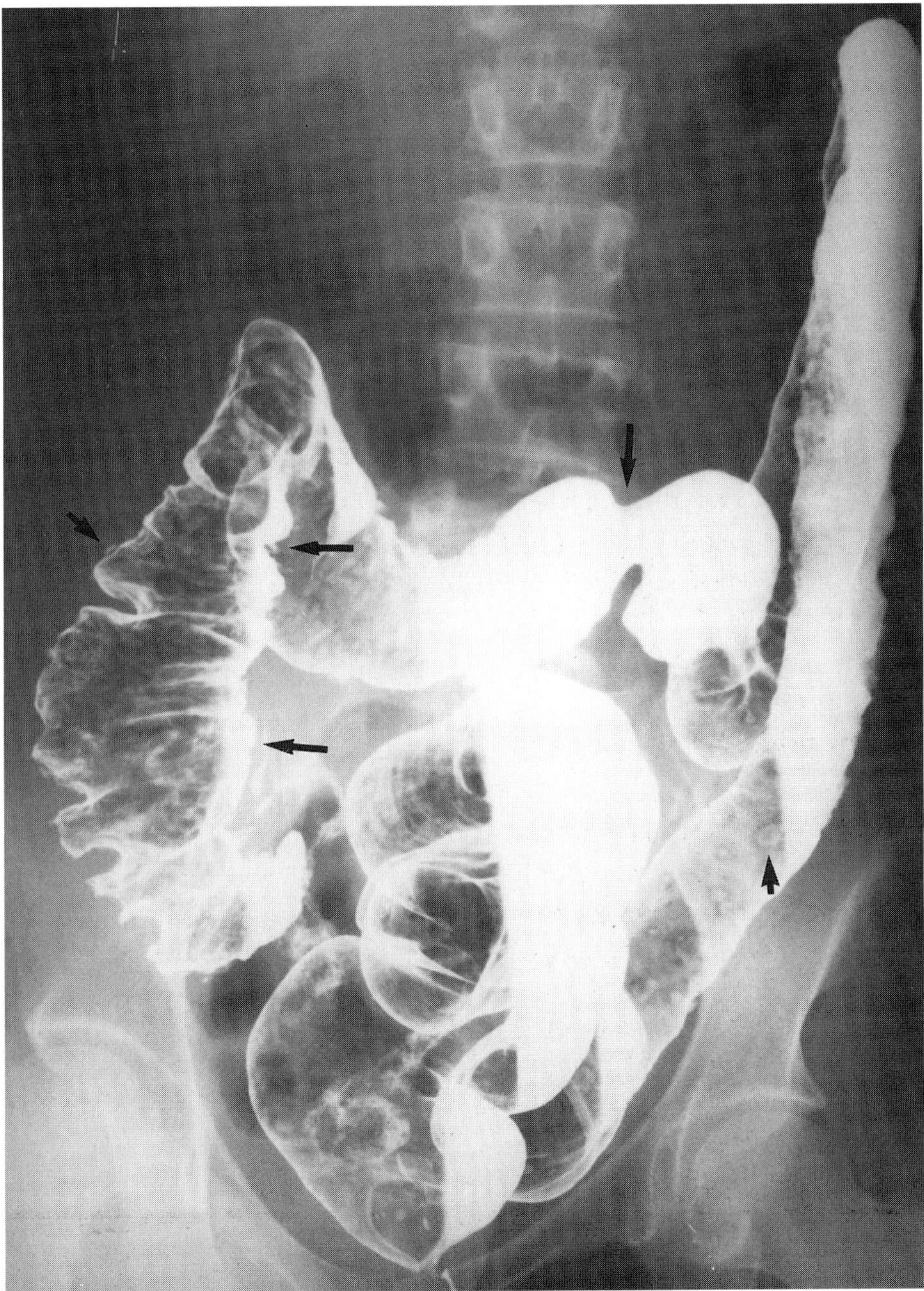

Figure 5.8.   Crohn's disease. 'Aphthous' ulcers. Stricture in transverse colon. Asymmetric involvement in ascending colon with loss of haustration and fibrosis on medial aspect. Note that 'collar stud' ulcers can also occur in Crohn's disease.

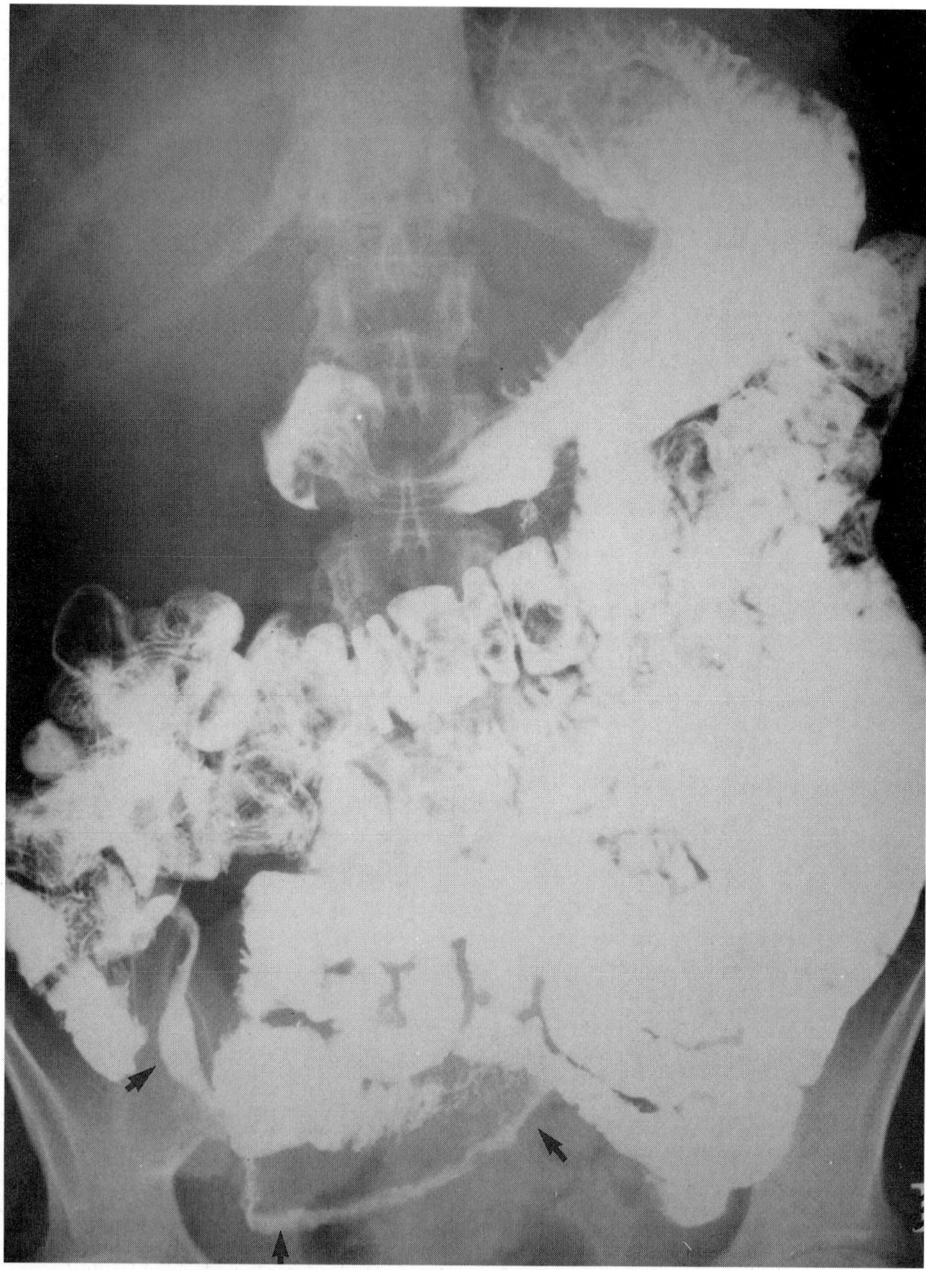

Figure 5.9.   Crohn's disease. 'String sign of Kantor': long narrowed segment of terminal ileum.

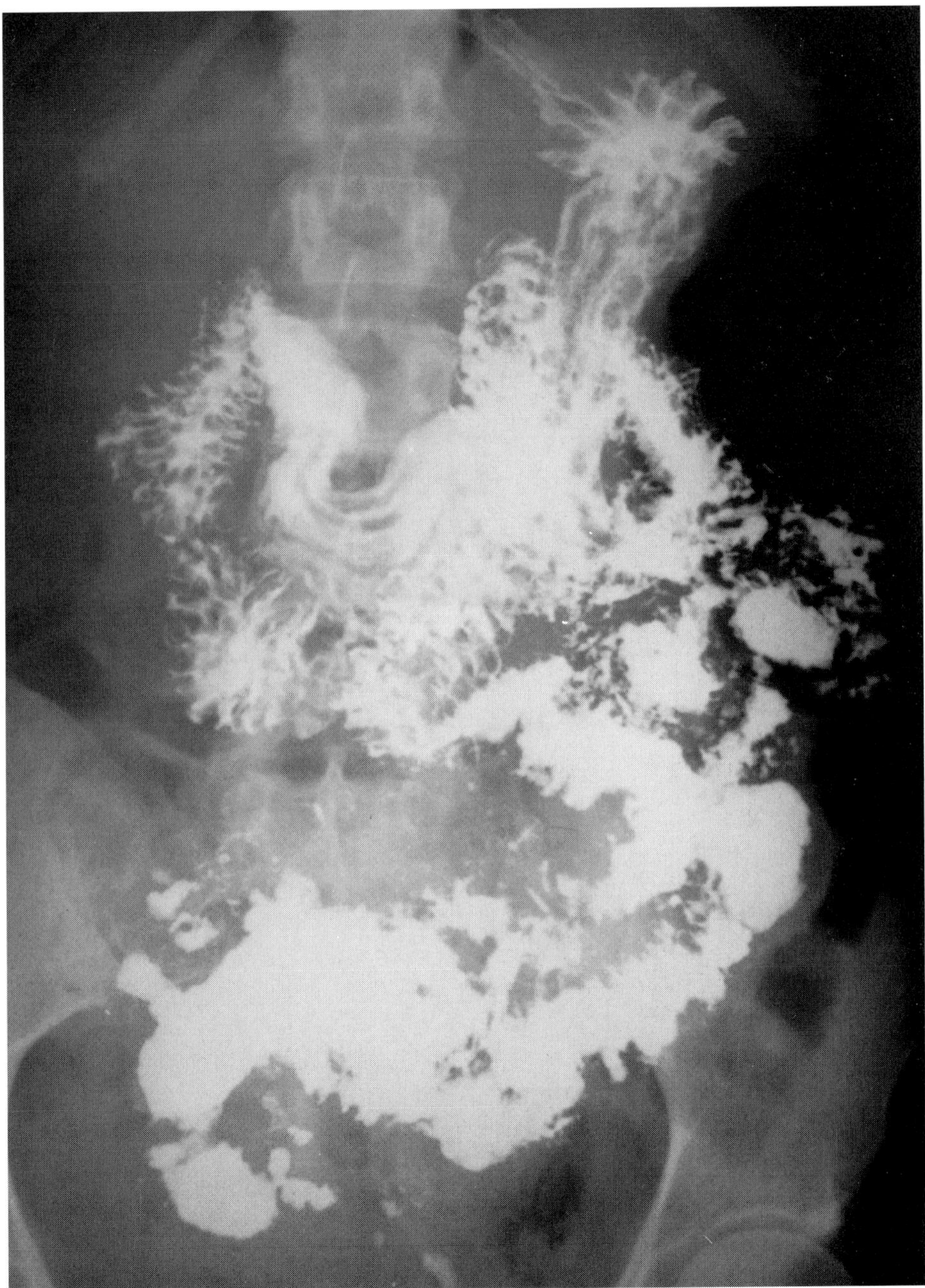

Figure 5.10. Malabsorption syndrome. Segmentation and dilatation of small bowel loops and flocculation and clumping of barium.

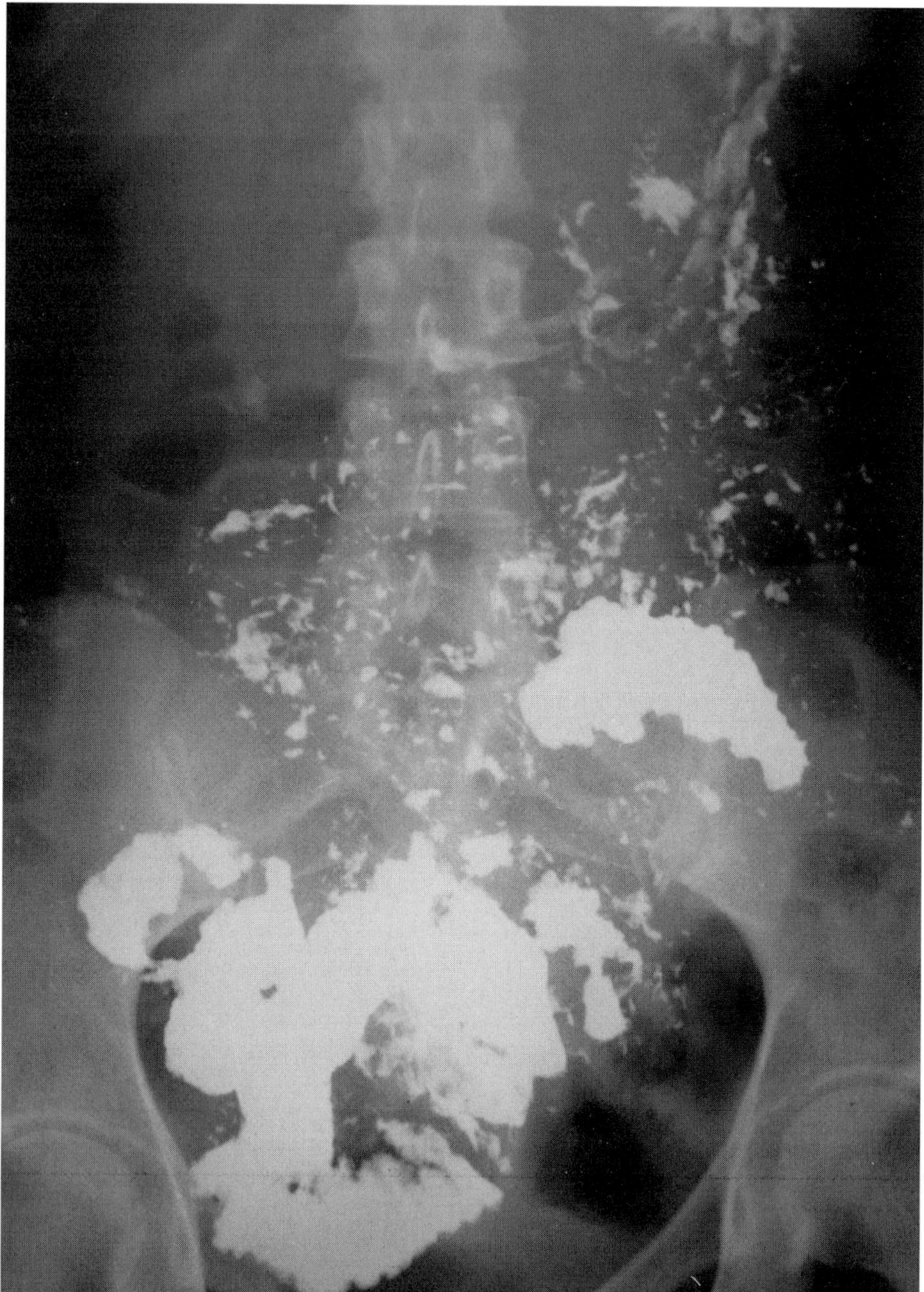

Figure 5.11. Malabsorption syndrome. Segmentation and dilatation of small bowel loops and flocculation and clumping of barium.

the bowel loops and fistulous communications with other loops. Skip lesions are common and, on occasions, there can be involvement of the stomach and duodenum. The other diseases that can mimic Crohn's disease are *Yersinia enterocolitica* infection and tuberculosis, especially when the involvement is in the ileocaecal region. Lymphosarcoma can produce similar appearances due to ulceration, thickening and blunting of the mucosal folds. The lumen is usually eccentric and intraluminal nodules are common. In Hodgkin's disease, there are multiple ulcerated filling defects with rigid areas devoid of mucosa. In scleroderma, the findings are of gross dilatation of the small bowel loops that are not thickened and there is no evidence of ulceration. There are multiple sites of functional obstruction due to lack of effective peristalsis.

Radiation enteritis produces severe oedema, ulceration and spasm (Figure 5.12).

Other abnormalities seen on barium follow-through are anatomical lesions of the small bowel due to previous resections, jejunal diverticulosis, stagnant loops, ileal strictures, fistulas and mixed lesions due to a combination of the above. In anatomical resections of the small bowel there is a rapid transit of small bowel contents resulting in malabsorption, although this is less common in jejunal resection than in ileal resection. Fistulas can short-circuit the gut causing intestinal hurry. An accurate interpretation of anatomical abnormalities seen after surgery on a barium meal follow-through examination requires accurate surgical detail. In intestinal tuberculosis the involvement of the small bowel is common, and strictures and matting of bowel loops are present.

In Zollinger–Ellison syndrome there is marked thickening of the gastric rugal folds, and single or multiple ulcers may be present in the stomach, duodenal bulb, duodenal loop or proximal small intestine. Eosinophilic gastroenteritis can produce thickening of the mucosal folds in the stomach and small bowel.

Other investigations

CT scanning of the abdomen could be of value in detection of lymphadenopathy in cancers, lymphoma and Whipple's disease. CT scanning, as well as ultrasound, can show metastatic disease of the liver or changes in the pancreas, as in chronic pancreatitis and pancreatic cancer. Mesenteric angiography may show areas of infarction in the bowel due to 'cut-off' of arterial supply.

In summary, in cases of adult diarrhoeal diseases, the radiological investigations help with the diagnosis. The choice of investigation depends upon the clinical features. Some clinical entities can be diagnosed by their characteristic radiological appearances, although there can often be considerable overlap and differentiation is not always easy. Plain x-rays are very helpful in the detection of pancreatic calcification and demonstration of toxic megacolon. Barium enema is usually

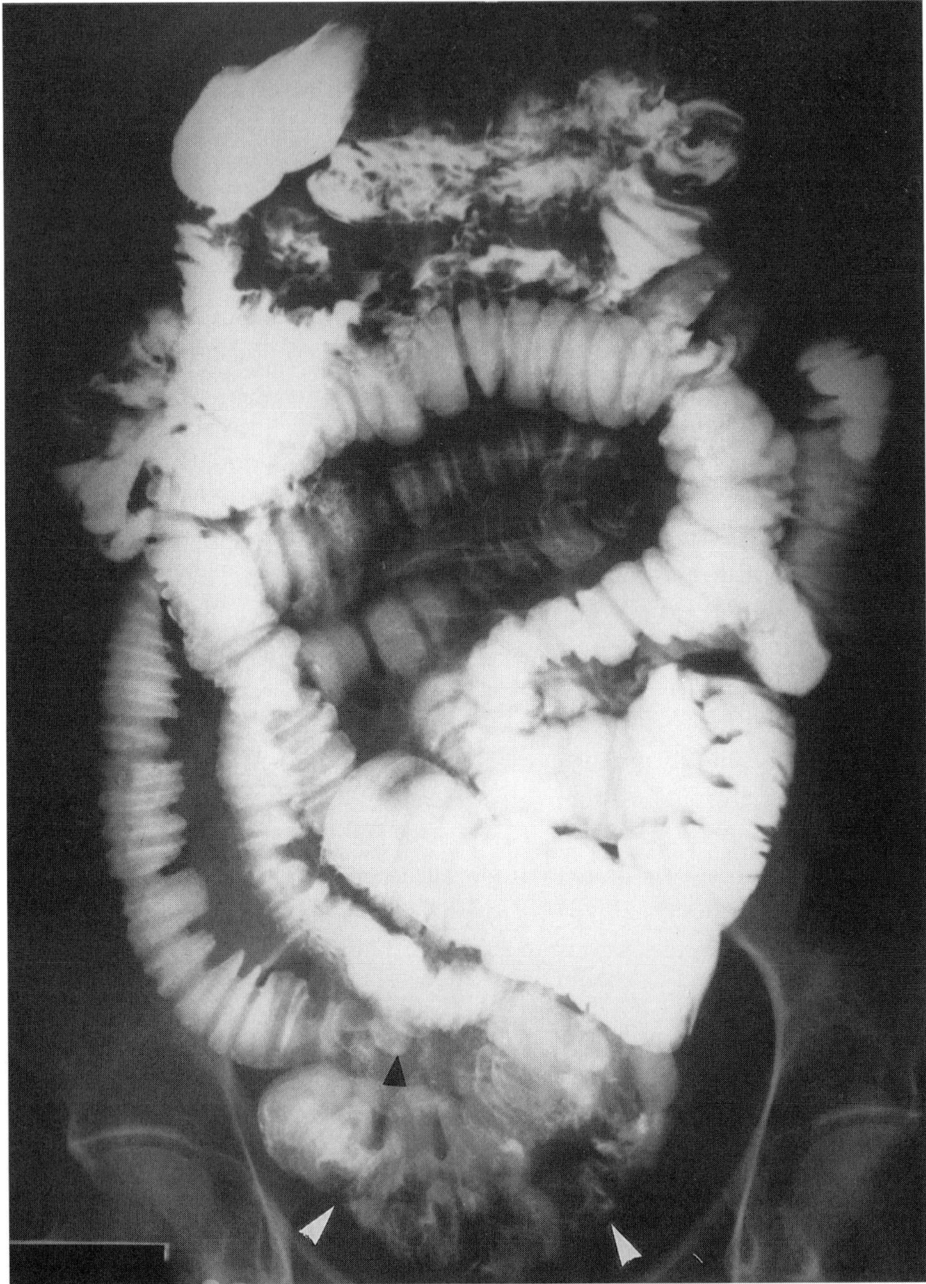

Figure 5.12. Radiation ileitis. Narrowing and marked mucosal oedema of the small bowel loops in the pelvis secondary to radiation therapy for carcinoma.

diagnostic in cases of Crohn's disease, ulcerative colitis, diverticular disease, ischaemic colitis and in the detection of cancers. Small bowel follow-through examinations are useful, though not diagnostic in malabsorption and in identifying anatomical abnormalities of the small intestine. CT and ultrasound examinations of the abdomen are occasionally required to supplement the diagnosis. Radiological investigations are not required in cases of acute infective, drug-induced diarrhoea, and diarrhoea due to metabolic causes.

BIBLIOGRAPHY AND FURTHER READING

Biochemical investigations

Dauterman, K.W., Bennett, R.G., Greenough, W.B. III et al. (1995). Plasma specific gravity for identifying hypovolaemia. *J. Diarrhoeal Dis. Res.* 13:33–8.

6 Faecal incontinence

Ludomyr J. Mykyta

Epidemiology

Faecal incontinence (FI) is a problem predominantly detected in the elderly and is particularly prevalent amongst institutionalized patients, unlike urinary incontinence, which occurs to a significant degree in all age groups. In nursing homes the prevalence is more than 20 per cent, usually in association with urinary incontinence, and is reported to range from 13 per cent to 47 per cent in hospitalized elderly patients. In residential homes in the United Kingdom (these homes provide a level of care that is approximately comparable to that offered in Australian hostels) the prevalence was 10.3 per cent. The prevalence of FI in a community setting was 10.9 per 1000 in males and 13.3 per 1000 in females over the age of 65 years.

Anorectal anatomy and physiology

The anal canal is surrounded by two concentric tubes of musculature, the internal and external sphincters (Figure 6.1). The internal sphincter is a thickened continuation of the rectal muscle wall, about 3 cm long and 4 mm deep, and is composed of smooth muscle. It is under autonomic control and accounts for 70 per cent of resting sphincter pressure.

The external sphincter, which constitutes the pelvic floor, is made up of striated muscle. The cranial part consists of the levator ani, the intermediate part is the puborectalis sling, and the caudal part is the external anal sphincter, which overlies the internal sphincter. Functionally, all of the components of the external sphincter act together.

The U-shaped puborectalis sling pulls the anorectal junction forward, causing occlusion of the anal canal by the anterior rectal wall (acting as a flap valve). The anorectal angle is normally maintained at about 80 degrees (range 60 to 105 degrees). During defaecation this angle is diminished by the relaxation of the puborectalis sling.

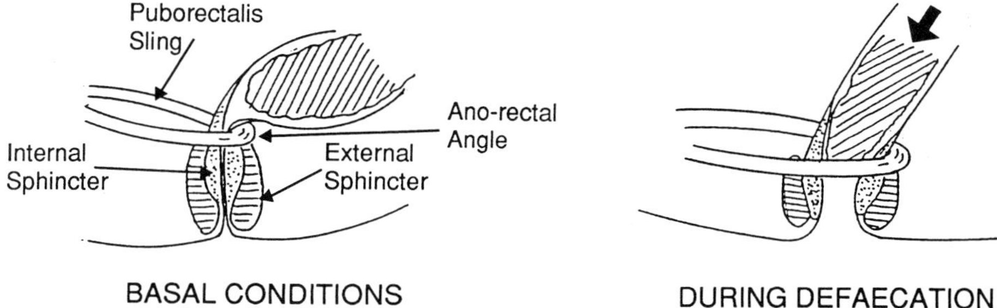

Figure 6.1.   The process of defaecation.

In the past, it was considered that this flap valve mechanism was the main means of maintaining continence. More recent radiological studies have raised doubts about its existence, and the success of surgical repair of the pelvic floor does not appear to rely on the restoration of the angle.

Anal closure is maintained by the continuous state of contraction of both the smooth and striated muscles. The latter is due to continuous reflex activity, which increases when intra-abdominal pressure rises (e.g. by coughing or straining) and ceases when defaecation is attempted.

Normally the resting pressure in the anal canal is between 70 and 100 cm of water which can be doubled temporarily by a voluntary contraction. Anal pressures (maximal anal squeeze) remain unchanged with age until the eighth decade in women and the ninth decade in men, after which they decline.

The sensory receptors responsible for the sensation of a full rectum are probably located in the pelvic floor musculature. Discrimination between flatus and faeces is probably carried out by a locally mediated reflex at the level of the anal canal. Suprasegmental and cortical control of faecal continence is not fully understood.

Distension of the rectum produces a desire to defaecate and causes reflex contraction of the rectal smooth muscle and relaxation of the internal anal sphincter. If the conditions are appropriate, the individual can initiate defaecation by contracting the abdominal muscles and diaphragm, and simultaneously relaxing the puborectalis and the external anal sphincter. If the situation is inappropriate, the contraction of the rectum and desire to defaecate can only be suppressed by strong contraction of the external sphincter and pushing of the stools back to the rectum.

Faecal continence requires:

- a suitable storage organ (adequate rectal distensibility)
- an appropriate consistency and volume of stool
- normal colonic transit time
- a functioning sphincter apparatus

Table 6.1. Causes of faecal incontinence

Faecal stasis	Bowel disorders	Neurological causes
Any cause of chronic constipation	• gastroenteritis • diverticulitis • irritable bowel syndrome • proctitis • rectal prolapse • perineal descent • fissure or fistula • carcinoma • megacolon • rectal or genital prolapse • diabetes mellitus • drugs • sphincter defect • trauma, any loss of anorectal angle • surgery	• dementia • acute confusion • spinal injury • 'idiopathic' • Parkinson's disease

- intact sensory function to sense rectal filling and to distinguish the nature of rectal contents
- adequate cognitive function to take appropriate actions
- adequate mobility and manual dexterity.

Pathophysiology and aetiological factors

The causes of FI are listed in Table 6.1.

In contrast to other age groups, constipation is the most common single cause of FI in institutionalized elderly people. The overflow of mucus and liquid stool around an impacted mass of faeces is called 'spurious diarrhoea'. The liquid stool creates a major risk to skin integrity and contributes significantly to the creation and perpetuation of pressure ulceration.

Constipation is a common problem in the elderly – and a frequent preoccupation. A review of the epidemiology of constipation in the USA found an overall prevalence of 2 per cent; that constipation increased with age, being most common after the age of 64 years; and that it was three times more common in women than in men. The review indicated that 45 per cent of elderly people use a laxative regularly.

While faecal impaction can cause a variety of clinical symptoms and signs, in institutionalized elderly people it frequently presents with paradoxical diarrhoea and incontinence, often double incontinence. Patients with faecal impaction have impaired anorectal sensation, and larger stool volumes are required than in controls to register awareness.

Constipation can be defined in terms of stool frequency, consistency and difficulty in evacuation. Ninety per cent of the population have a bowel frequency of between three motions per day and three motions per week. It is generally accepted that constipation is present when bowel frequency is less than three times per week. Patients with constipation may also complain of hard and dry (usually associated with decreased frequency) stool or painful or difficult stool.

In summary, constipation is not a disease, but a symptom which may be:

- due to organic disease of the anus, rectum or colon
- secondary to systemic disease (see Chapter 16) or drugs (see Chapter 7)

Other causes of faecal incontinence

Faecal incontinence in patients with weakness of the sphincter muscles without an apparent cause has been termed 'idiopathic', although there is usually evidence that the nerve supply of the striated sphincter (pudendal nerves and direct branches of the sacral motor nerve roots) is damaged. This damage may occur due to stretching during childbirth or excessive prolonged straining at stool because of chronic constipation.

Patient evaluation

History

Past and general history should cover the presence of diabetes mellitus, neurological disorders and medication use. In women, obstetric history and any pelvic surgery should be considered. Bowel history should include previous bowel disorders or bowel surgery. The frequency and severity of the incontinence should be documented. Incontinence can be partial or complete. Partial incontinence involves the passage of flatus and some faecal soiling, and often occurs only in the presence of loose stool. Complete incontinence is defined as the frequent and regular deficiency in the ability to control stool of normal consistency.

Constipation and faecal impaction are frequently accompanied by a variety of symptoms that include abdominal bloating, discomfort and pain which may be colicky and quite severe, anorexia, nausea, malaise and headache. The patient may be confused and restless.

Clinical examination

A complete physical examination with particular emphasis on neurological examination should be carried out in all patients. Rectal examination is essential.

Normally the anus is closed and when the perianal skin is stimulated the external anal sphincter visibly contracts (the anal reflex). The anal verge is located below a line drawn from the tip of the coccyx to the inferior margin of the symphysis pubis. The perineal level should not descend more than 2 cm when the patient is asked to strain.

With digital examination it is possible to feel the anal resting tone and the voluntary contraction of the sphincter on voluntary contraction or on coughing (the cough reflex). The puborectalis sling can be felt as a posterior ring of muscle at the level of the upper anal canal. An empty rectum does not rule out the possibility of faecal impaction. High impactions are not uncommon and the presence of a high impaction raises the suspicion of a colonic carcinoma. Clinical examination may include proctoscopy and sigmoidoscopy.

Patients with central neurological causes exhibit a type of faecal incontinence that is analogous to the uninhibited bladder. They are unable to inhibit defaecation and pass formed stools into the bed or clothing.

Investigation

Investigation will be dictated by the clinical picture and may include plain x-ray of the abdomen, barium enema or colonoscopy. A plain x-ray of the abdomen is useful in diagnosing high faecal impaction when the rectum is empty.

A technique of using pelvic ultrasound to determine the anorectal angle and puborectalis function has been described. This has the advantage of not exposing the patient to radiation.

Anal ultrasonography allows accurate definition of defects in the internal and external sphincters and provides a qualitative assessment of the muscle. This has altered the understanding of faecal incontinence, as well as its investigation and management. Such studies have shown a high incidence of structural defects affecting the sphincters, and therefore cast some doubt on the overall importance of neurological factors in the pathogenesis of faecal incontinence.

Anal function can be investigated specifically by manometry and electromyography. This type of investigation is generally confined to research centres rather than being a regular part of the physician's armamentarium.

Management

Conservative management of constipation

Faecal impaction and overflow is most commonly managed by disimpaction and complete bowel clearance, and a preventive regime of bowel care.

Manual disimpaction is usually required at the outset, particularly if the faecal mass is hard and dry. Local anaesthetic jelly can be used to lubricate the glove. If carried out carefully the procedure can be performed without undue distress.

Once fragmentation has been achieved, clearance is continued with enemas.

Table 6.2. Selected dietary items with a high fibre content

Source	Serve	Fibre per serve (g)
Fruit		
Dried fruit, average	30 g	5.0
Apple – fresh, with skin	150 g	4.5
Figs	100 g (2 large)	4.0
Grains and cereals		
All Bran	30 g	9.3
Muesli	Average serve	8.0
Wholemeal roll	1 roll	5.1
Vita-Brits	32 g (2 biscuits)	3.6
Pasta	Average serve	3.5
Unprocessed bran	1 tsp	3.0
Legumes		
Red kidney beans (cooled)	100 g	7.4
Baked beans	100 g	7.3
Vegetables		
Peas, canned	1/2 cup	6.7
Spinach	60 g	4.0
Potato, with skin	100 g	3.5
Broccoli	1/2 cup	3.5
Corn	1/2 ear	2.6

These are administered daily or twice daily until the bowel is cleared. This may take several days as the whole colon may be loaded.

A stepped-care approach to chronic constipation

1.   Utilize times of high bowel motility, which are on rising and after meals. Encourage the patient to develop a good bowel habit by responding to the call to stool that occurs at these times.

2.   Increase dietary fibre and fluid intake. Not all fruits and vegetables are rich sources of fibre (Table 6.2). Fibre should be introduced gradually as many patients complain of early bloating. The recommended intake of fibre is approximately 30–35 g/day. The aim is to convert a small stool that sinks to a bulky stool that floats.

     Fluid intake should be at least 1.5 l/day. Patients find it helpful if this is translated into an easily understood quantity.

     If these measures are insufficient, hydrophilic colloids can be added, e.g Agiofibe, Fybogel, Granocol, Metamucil or Normacol. Most are taken as one to two teaspoonsful (5–10 g) once or twice daily after the main meal or on retiring. It is very important to maintain an adequate fluid intake when using these agents. They have the potential to increase constipation if the fluid intake is inadequate.

A study undertaken at the Phillip Kennedy Center in Adelaide, South Australia, demonstrated that the planned use of dietary fibre and a controlled fluid intake could almost eliminate the need for aperients while restoring bowel function in nursing-home patients.

3. Add a stool softener, dioctyl sodium sulfosuccinate (Coloxyl) 120 mg, two tablets after the evening meal. It may cause mucosal damage and should not be used in the long term.

    The vegetable root preparation 'Nu-Lax' may be tried at this stage. Its mode of action is unclear, but it appears to be safe for long-term use.

4. If there is no response, try an irritant (stimulant) agent, e.g. bisacodyl (Bisalax, Durolax), one to three tablets, in the evening. These drugs should be used only occasionally, e.g. once or twice weekly.

5. Introduce an osmotic laxative. These agents are safe and are suitable for long-term use, e.g. lactulose (Duphalac) or sorbitol (Sorbilax) 10–45 ml as a single daily dose after breakfast.

6. Local agents (enemas and suppositories) act by distending the rectum and colon and stimulating a reflex evacuation.

Prevention of constipation

Prevention relies on the adequate management of constipation. Patients should be encouraged to modify their diets to include an adequate amount of vegetable fibre, and an adequate fluid intake. They should exercise regularly, develop a regular bowel habit and avoid reliance on, and protracted use of, laxatives.

Management of faecal incontinence

A variety of approaches is available to manage faecal incontinence in the absence of faecal impaction. A conservative approach will achieve continence in most elderly patients. With mild degrees of incontinence a high fibre diet, or a bulking agent, or both, can be used to produce stool of more manageable consistency. Biofeedback training, using a balloon to simulate rectal distension by stool, and training the patient to decrease the threshold of rectal sensation to distension to contract the anal sphincter voluntarily in response to this stimulus, has been reported as highly successful by some authors. Patient selection is based on motivation, capacity to comprehend instructions, and intact rectal sensation. Biofeedback training is therefore most probably suitable for younger patients. In some patients with long-established denervation a regime of constipation and planned evacuation may be employed. The commonly used agents include loperamide (Imodium), which not only enhances faecal consistency but also increases anal sphincter pressure.

Where conservative management is unsuccessful, it will be necessary to use an appropriate pad system. There are a large variety of pads on the market and advice about the suitability of a particular product can be obtained from experienced nurses.

Anal plugs have been on trial with success and may prove to have a significant place in management.

Surgery

Surgery for faecal incontinence is rarely performed on elderly patients, in part because of the likelihood that the problem can be managed conservatively, and in part because of the coexistence of other problems, particularly dementia, which complicate the clinical picture and increase surgical risk.

The clearest indication for a surgical repair is severe faecal incontinence with evidence of sphincter damage. Where the sphincter has been severed, it can be repaired directly. If there is neurological damage, postanal repair can be carried out. The success rates are of the order of 60–70 per cent. Surgery in patients with neurological damage is usually not very successful. In rectal prolapse, the most successful operations appear to require an abdominal approach.

BIBLIOGRAPHY AND FURTHER READING

Barrett, J.A., Brocklehurst, J.C., Kiff, E.S., Ferguson, G. & Faragher, E.B. (1989). Anal function in geriatric patients with faecal incontinence. *Gut* **30**:1244–51.

Bartolo, D.C. (1991). Gastroenterological options in faecal incontinence. *Ann. Chir.* **45**:590–8.

Castle, S.C. (1989). Constipation: endemic in the elderly? Gerontopathophysiology, evaluation and management. *Med. Clin. N. Am.* **73**:1497–509.

Corman, M.L. (1983). The management of anal incontinence. *Surg. Clin. N. Am.* **63**:177–92.

Goldstein, M.K., Brown, E.M., Holt, P., Gallagher, D. & Winograd, C.H. (1989). Fecal incontinence in an elderly man. Stanford University Geriatrics Case Conference. *J. Am. Geriatr. Soc.* **37**:991–1002.

Henry, M.M. (1987). Pathogenesis and management of fecal incontinence in the adult. *Gastroenterol. Clin. N. Am.* **16**:35–45.

Hope, A.K. & Down, E.C. (1986). Dietary fibre and fluid in the control of constipation in a nursing home population. *Med. J. Aust.* **144**:306–7.

Loening-Baucke, V. (1990). Efficacy of biofeedback training in improving faecal incontinence and anorectal physiologic function. *Gut* **31**:1395–402.

Madoff, R.D., Williams, J.G. & Caushaj, P.F. (1992). Fecal incontinence. *N. Engl. J. Med.* **326**:1002–7.

Mortensen, N. & Humphreys, M.S. (1991). The anal continence plug: a disposable device for patients with anorectal incontinence. *Lancet* **338**:295–7.

Pittman, J.S., Benson, J.T. & Sumners, J.E. (1990). Physiologic evaluation of the anorectum. A new ultrasound technique. *Dis. Colon Rectum* **33**:476–8.

Read, M. & Read, N.W. (1982). Effects of loperamide on anal sphincter function in patients complaining of chronic diarrhoea with faecal incontinence and urgency. *Dig. Dis. Sci.* **27**:807–14.

Read, N.W. & Abouzekry, L. (1986). Why do patients with faecal impaction have faecal incontinence. *Gut* **27**:283–7.

Smith, R.G. (1990). Large bowel problems. *Br. Med. Bull.* **46**:246–61.

Sun, W.M., Donnelly, T.C. & Read, N.W. (1992). Utility of combined test of anorectal manometry, electromyography, and sensation in determining the mechanism of 'idiopathic' faecal incontinence. *Gut* **33**:807–13.

Thomas, T.M., Egan, M., Walgrove, A. & Meade, T.W. (1984). The prevalence of faecal and double incontinence. *Community Med.* **6**:216–20.

Tobin, G.W. & Brocklehurst, J.C. (1986). Faecal incontinence in residential homes for the elderly: prevalence, aetiology and management. *Age Ageing* **15**: 41–6.

Wald, A. (1990). Constipation and fecal incontinence in the elderly. *Gastroenterol Clin. N. Am.* **19**:405–18.

Wexner, S.D., Marchetti, F. & Jagelman, D.G. (1991). The role of sphincteroplasty for fecal incontinence reevaluated: a prospective physiologic and functional review. *Dis. Colon Rectum* **34**:22–30.

Whitehead, W.E., Drinkwater, D., Cheskin, L.J., Heller, B.R. & Schuster, M.M. (1989). Constipation in the elderly living at home. Definition, prevalence, and relationship to lifestyle and health status. *J. Am. Geriatr. Soc.* **37**:423–9.

Wrenn, K. (1989). Fecal impaction. *New Engl. J. Med.* **321**:658–62.

Wunderlich, M. & Parks, A.G. (1982). Physiology and pathophysiology of the anal sphincters. *Int. Surg.* **67**:291–8.

7 Drug-induced diarrhoea

Ranjit N. Ratnaike and Terry E. Jones

Introduction

Diarrhoea is a problem in the elderly population where a significant and major cause is the adverse effects of drugs. Drug consumption increases with age, being highest in the elderly, affluent, white female patient, and amplifies the potential for adverse drug reactions and drug–drug interactions. In addition, the elderly patient is more likely to suffer from the adverse effects of drugs (including diarrhoea) due to blunted homeostatic mechanisms and impaired drug handling.

The elderly are an increasing portion of the total population and they consume a disproportionately large number of drugs; this disparity is in part due to the vast number of drugs now available to treat diseases associated with old age. Most drugs consumed by the elderly are for chronic conditions and therefore therapy is often for prolonged periods. It is likely that adverse effects and/or interactions, including drug-associated diarrhoea, will increase in frequency.

The number of diseases for which drug interventions are available increases with greater knowledge of the disease processes and the advent of new diagnostic tools. New classes of drugs have become available for managing myocardial ischaemia and cardiac failure, hypertension, peptic ulcer and reflux oesophagitis. These drugs include the angiotensin–converting enzyme inhibitors (ACEIs) (e.g. captopril and enalapril), HMG–CoA–reductase inhibitors (e.g. atorvastatin, pravastatin, lovostatin and simvastatin), and inhibitors of gastric acid production (e.g. ranitidine and omeprazole).

In Western countries, because of the ability of consumers to pay for new drugs, research into the diseases which afflict the elderly continues and is likely to expand. This contrasts with the limited research into diseases which are prevalent in developing countries where, due to lack of funds, older, more toxic agents are often all that can be afforded by the majority of people. Poor regulation of drug availability in many developing countries compounds the problem.

Drug consumption by various groups of elderly people has been investigated by several authors (Table 7.1). Often these data exclude 'over-the-counter' drugs (including 'herbal remedies'), many of which cause diarrhoea (e.g. antacids and

Table 7.1. Frequency of drug consumption in the elderly

Drug type	Frequency of use (%)
NSAIDs	15.0 – 45.0
Cardiac glycosides	6.0–60.0
Diuretics	12.0–36.0
Analgesics	6.0–17.0
Cardiovascular	10.0–73.0
Psychotropic	6.5–57.0
Gastrointestinal	3.5–18.5

laxatives). The drugs most commonly associated with diarrhoea are listed below:

- antibiotics – especially clindamycin and ampicillin
- antimetabolites – fluorouracil, methotrexate
- cardiovascular agents – methyldopa, digitalis, quinidine, propranolol, amiloride, bretylium, guanethidine, triamterene
- gastrointestinal agents – laxatives, misoprostol, lactulose, antacids (Mg salts), H_2 receptor antagonists, cholestyramine, acarbose, chenodeoxycholic acid, olsalazine
- musculoskeletal agents – colchicine, indomethacin, auranofin, naproxen, phenylbutazone, mefenamic acid, diflunisal
- central nervous system drugs – anticholinergic agents, levodopa, alprazolam, lithium, meprobamate
- genitourinary system drugs – propantheline
- miscellaneous drugs – metformin, gastrografin, clofibrate, iron (this usually causes constipation, but diarrhoea can occur).

The pathophysiology underlying drug-induced diarrhoea is established in many instances while, with others, the mechanism is yet to be determined.

Drugs may cause diarrhoea in a variety of ways including: impairing either immune defences or nonimmune defences, or interfering with mechanisms of normal fluid absorption and secretion. Sometimes more than one mechanism may be involved, as with auranofin the oral gold preparation, olsalazine used in ulcerative colitis, and the synthetic prostaglandin analogues misoprostol and enprostil as discussed below.

Immune mechanisms

The production of secretory IgA, the primary immune response of the gastrointestinal tract, is highly T-cell (particularly T_4) dependent. Aging results in a decrease in both the quality and proportion of T-helper and T-suppressor subpopulations. T-cell numbers and function can be further impaired by drugs which compromise the immune system, thereby increasing host susceptibility to intestinal infections.

Nonimmune defences

The nonimmunological defences include the gastric acid barrier, motility of the small intestine, and the commensal bacteria of the large intestine.

Gastric acid secretion

Gastric acid production is an important line of defence against pathogens which have the ability to cause diarrhoea (see Chapter 1). Almost 80 per cent of otherwise healthy octogenarians were shown to be hypochlorhydric and to have microbial colonization. Drugs can reduce the production of, or neutralize, gastric acid, thereby impairing this protective mechanism.

The treatment of peptic ulcer disease and/or reflux oesophagitis usually involves drugs which reduce acid production, and this is particularly relevant in the elderly. Cimetidine, an H_2 receptor blocker, causes diarrhoea in 3 to 12 per cent of patients and is a significant risk factor for the carriage of *Clostridium difficile*, with the potential to develop pseudomembraneous colitis. Omeprazole, the powerful proton pump inhibitor, resulted in bacterial overgrowth in 53 per cent of patients.

Transient, dose-related diarrhoea and abdominal cramping are the most common adverse effects of misoprostol (a synthetic analogue of prostaglandin E), which inhibits gastric acid and pepsin production.

Intestinal motility

Normal intestinal motility associated with the migrating motor complex (MMC) transports digested food products, removes the continuously replenished mucus layer and prevents prolonged contact between enteric pathogens, toxins, and the small bowel mucosa. In the elderly – uniquely – despite normal anatomy of the small intestine and no obvious localized or systemic cause, hypomotility and bacterial overgrowth are well established.

In bacterial overgrowth, diarrhoea is due to bacterial deconjugation of primary bile salts to dihydroxy bile acids (predominantly deoxycholic acid) which effect net fluid and electrolyte secretion in the colon. Bile salt deconjugation also impairs micelle formation and may lead to steatorrhoea.

Diarrhoea due to drug-induced hypermotility is uncommon. Tacrine, a cholinesterase inhibitor used in Alzheimer's disease, can cause diarrhoea which is the most severe clinical side effect due to its cholinergic action. Irinotecan, a new agent in treating colorectal cancer, causes severe diarrhoea due to a cholinergic-like syndrome by inhibition of acetylcholinesterase.

Intestinal motility can be impaired by drugs. Iatrogenic reduction of intestinal motility from anticholinergic drug use facilitates bacterial overgrowth. Diarrhoea occurs due to bacterial enzymatic deconjugation of primary bile salts to dihydroxy bile acids (predominantly deoxycholic acid). Another consequence of bile salt deconjugation is impairment of micelle formation resulting in steatorrhea.

Anticholinergic drugs which were extensively used for the treatment of peptic ulcer disease are now superseded by more effective agents. Other drugs with anticholinergic activity include propantheline (prescribed for the treatment of urinary incontinence), benztropine (prescribed for Parkinson's disease), and tricyclic antidepressants. Despite their potential to cause diarrhoea, anticholinergic drugs more often cause constipation. However, these drugs should be considered as possible contributory factors if the aetiology of diarrhoea is obscure in the elderly patient.

Intestinal flora

The micro-organisms of the large intestine are an important defence protecting the host from harmful pathogens and, consequently, diarrhoea. These commensal bacteria form a complex, well balanced ecological system to defend the host by mechanisms such as modification of bile acids; stimulation of peristalsis; induction of immunological responses; depletion of essential substrates from the environment; competition for adhesion sites; creation of restrictive metabolic environments; and elaboration of antibiotic-like substances.

Drugs can impair this nonimmune defence. Antibiotics, especially those with a broad spectrum of activity, kill large numbers of intestinal bacteria and, due to their extensive use, are the most frequent iatrogenic causes of diarrhoea in the elderly.

The most common form of drug-induced diarrhoea is pseudomembraneous colitis, a suprainfection caused by *Clostridium difficile*. This anaerobe is normally unable to colonize the gastrointestinal tract due to competition from the normal commensal population. A decrease in colonic bacterial numbers after antibiotic administration can result in *C. difficile* overgrowth.

Most antibiotics have been implicated, particularly clindamycin, although amoxycillin and ampicillin are often involved due to their frequent use. Recently, cephalosporins have been increasingly implicated in *C. difficile* diarrhoea. Suprainfection by *C. difficile* can present as a self-limiting illness with only mild diarrhoea or as a more severe syndrome of pseudomembraneous colitis.

Those at risk of acquiring *C. difficile* are the elderly in hospitals and long-term care patients, and those on chemotherapy for malignancy. The incidence of *C. difficile* infections is increased by the presence of feeding tubes, urinary and faecal incontinence, and when three or more underlying diseases are present.

Treatment with antibiotics in mild cases may not be necessary. In the elderly, appropriate guidelines for antibiotic use would be: 5–6 bowel motions within 24 hours, diarrhoea persisting for more than 48 hours, blood in the stools, dehydration, evidence of fever, abdominal pain or tenderness, rectal pain or tenesmus, or the patient having multiple medical problems.

Oral vancomycin, bacitracin or metronidazole are the drugs of choice. While vancomycin may be more efficacious than metronidazole, the latter should be the agent of first choice because of concerns over the recent emergence of vancomycin-resistant enterococci. Vancomycin must be administered orally as it is not secreted into the gut, but should be reserved for unresponsive or relapsing cases. Instances of relapse are not uncommon and, in such cases, vancomycin should be administered for two weeks, while other measures such as hand washing and ward cleaning should be reviewed. Vancomycin and metronidazole have been previously shown to have equivalent efficacy and relapse rates, but the cost of metronidazole is significantly less.

Other suprainfections that lead to diarrhoea after antibiotic therapy are due to *C. perfringens*, *Salmonella* and *Shigella*.

Impairment of fluid absorption

Drugs can interrupt the normal processes of active and passive fluid and electrolyte absorption and secretion throughout the intestine (see Chapter 3).

In drug-induced secretory diarrhoea, the drug binds to a specific receptor on the cell surface and activates an internal enzyme system which activates adenylate cyclase and increases the concentration of cAMP. This results in the active secretion of anions (Cl and HCO_3), the passive efflux of Na, K and water and the inhibition of Na and Cl into the cell.

Misoprostol, dihydroxy bile acids (the end products of bacterial deconjugation of primary bile salts) and chenodeoxycholic acid (used in the dissolution of cholesterol gall stones) cause diarrhoea in this way. Ricinoleic acid (the end product of castor oil hydrolysis by colonic bacteria) and common laxatives such as dioctyl sodium sulphosuccinate and bisacodyl, cause diarrhoea through a similar process.

Drugs also interfere with the Na–K exchange pump, a second physiological system that regulates transport of water and electrolytes and hence intestinal secretory activity at the cellular level. The energy for this pump is provided by the breakdown of ATP, mediated via ATPase. The drugs mentioned below affect this Na–K exchange pump, thereby reducing fluid absorption which may result in diarrhoea.

Digoxin was second to antibiotics as the most common cause of diarrhoea in a study of 100 elderly inpatients. Digoxin is almost completely absorbed from the small intestine, but small amounts reach the colon where it interferes with ATPase activity, effecting a net fluid secretion. Diarrhoea is more likely to occur when blood levels exceed the normal therapeutic range. Digoxin is primarily excreted via the kidneys and, since renal function declines with age, digoxin-induced diarrhoea is more likely to occur in the elderly.

Diarrhoea is a well described side effect of auranofin, an oral gold preparation used in rheumatoid arthritis. Auranofin causes a concentration-dependent inhibition of ATPase activity.

The long-term administration of colchicine in smaller doses (1.0–2.0 mg/day) to patients with recurrent polyserositis (familial Mediterranean fever), is associated with diarrhoea. The mechanism of diarrhoea is inhibition of ATPase activity within the intestine epithelial cells.

Olsalazine is a relatively new, sulfa-free form of 5–aminosalicylate (5–ASA) used in the treatment of ulcerative colitis. Colonic bacterial metabolism liberates 5–aminosalicylate to the large intestine with minimal systemic absorption. Diarrhoea is a side effect reported in 10–25 per cent of patients. The drug causes a concentration-dependent inhibition of Na–K ATPase. This inhibits the ileal and colonic Na–K pump (see Chapter 3) and the consequent decreased fluid absorption leads to diarrhoea.

Drug-induced osmotic diarrhoea

The presence of osmotically active substances within the gastrointestinal tract decreases fluid absorption into the bloodstream. Compound antacid preparations attempt to balance the constipative effects of the aluminium component with the diarrhoeal effect of magnesium. Inevitably the constipative or laxative effect will predominate in a few patients. Diarrhoea occurs in a significant number of patients on antacids containing magnesium trisilicate or hydroxide and is dose dependent.

Lactulose, sorbitol and Epsom salts act osmotically within the colon to produce diarrhoea. Lactulose is a synthetic disaccharide which was initially used in the treatment of constipation but is now also used extensively in the treatment of hepatic encephalopathy and in the long-term management of patients with decompensated liver disease to improve protein tolerance. Since it is a synthetic disaccharide, lactulose is not affected by the small intestinal disaccharidases and therefore reaches the colon unchanged. Here, lactulose is metabolized by colonic bacteria to simple acids which exert an osmotic action in the colon.

Acarbose, the first of a new group of agents that improves blood sugar control is another drug which causes osmotic diarrhoea. Acarbose inhibits the action of intestinal alpha glucosidase which breaks down carbohydrate to monosaccharide in the gastrointestinal tract. In the colon the accumulated undigested, nonabsorbed carbohydrate is fermented and often leads to diarrhoea and flatulence. Propranolol, although an infrequent cause of diarrhoea, has been reported to cause an osmotic diarrhoea.

Mucosal damage

Drugs can cause diarrhoea by direct damage to the small intestinal mucosa. The clinical picture is one of malabsorption with bulky, foul smelling stools that are difficult to flush. Small bowel biopsy on patients and volunteers given neomycin shows varying degrees of histological change from loss of only microvilli to severe villous atrophy. Large doses of colchicine used in the treatment of gout cause villous atrophy, malabsorption and diarrhoea.

Similarly, antineoplastic drugs can cause diarrhoea by damaging immature epithelial cells in the crypt, resulting in the subsequent mature enterocytes being functionally compromised, decreasing their absorptive capacity and leading to diarrhoea.

Diarrhoea can also occur as a result of colitis. In addition to antibiotics, the better known drugs which cause colitis are: gold salts (including auranofin), antimetabolite cancer chemotherapeutic agents, penicillamine, methyldopa and the nonsteroidal antiinflammatory agents. With auranofin the colitis may persist despite withdrawal of the drug.

Laxative abuse

Definitions of diarrhoea and constipation are not easy to find for the public. What constitutes a normal bowel action reflects a perceived notion which may be highly individualistic, based on frequency and consistency of motions. The elderly tend to focus on this aspect of daily life and are more likely to resort to pharmacological intervention to restore bowel function to what is perceived as 'normal'. Laxatives intended for the acute relief of an episode of constipation may continue to be used and not mentioned during history taking in patients who are unaware of the nature of the medication.

The problem of surreptitious laxative abuse has been documented in the elderly and should be considered particularly in elderly female patients presenting with diarrhoea of an elusive aetiology. The surreptitious use of laxatives was found to be the cause of diarrhoea in 15–20 per cent of individuals who presented for investigation to a tertiary referral centre. In one study from the USA, in 20 of 67 patients who underwent extensive investigations for diarrhoea, laxative abuse was the most common cause. Patients may present with a variety of eating or psychiatric disorders and will usually deny laxative use. Screening for laxative use (either on stool water or urine) is often overlooked but is important since some patients will continue to use laxatives even after admission to hospital. Screening tests may include thin layer chromatography to detect anthroquinones, bisacodyl and phenolphthalein, stool osmolality to detect osmotically active laxatives and/or stool phosphate or sulphate concentration. These tests will also detect those individuals who alter the composition of their stool specimens by adding fluid to the stool sample

The elderly are especially susceptible to the adverse effects of drugs including diarrhoea, both as a consequence of the aging process and increased drug consumption.

The elderly patient often may not be aware of the reason for taking each of the drugs that are prescribed. Information about the adverse effects and uses of drugs is frequently not given to patients. The elderly are especially vulnerable since many have difficulty reading written information due to failing eyesight or severe dementia. Verbal information may not be retained due to impaired memory. In practice many elderly patients continue to take drugs which cause significant adverse effects including diarrhoea because they do not associate the adverse effect with the drug. Herbal remedies should not be overlooked as causes of diarrhoea.

In the context of diarrhoea in the elderly, the common problem of 'overflow diarrhoea', also known as 'spurious diarrhoea', a consequence of constipation, should be considered before a diagnosis of 'true diarrhoea' is made (see Chapter 6).

When an elderly person presents with diarrhoea, careful questioning of the patient may reveal a drug-related cause; often, however, more information may have to be sought from relatives, carers and the patient's physician or pharmacist. The practice of sighting all drugs the patient uses has much to be commended. This simple exercise, so often overlooked, accompanied by a detailed history would avoid many of the unnecessary, uncomfortable and expensive investigations undertaken to determine the cause of diarrhoea.

BIBLIOGRAPHY AND FURTHER READING

Ammon, H.V., Fowle, S.A., Cunningham, J.A., Komorowski, R.A. & Loeffler, R.F. (1987). Effect of auranofin and myochrysine on intestinal transport and morphology in the rat. *Gut* 28:829–34.

Andrejak, M., Schmit, J.L. & Tondriaux, A. (1991). The clinical significance of antibiotic-associated pseudomembranous colitis in the 1990s. *Drug Saf.* 6:339–49.

Bennett, G.C., Allen, E. & Millard, P.H. (1984). *Clostridium difficile* diarrhoea: a highly infectious organism. *Age Ageing* 13:363–6.

Bytzer, P., Stokholm, M., Andersen, I., Klitgaard, N.A. & Schafflitzky-de-Muckadell, O.B. (1989). Prevalence of surreptitious laxative abuse in patients with diarrhoea of uncertain origin: a cost benefit analysis of a screening procedure. *Gut* 10:1379–84.

Chawla, A., Karl, P.I., Riech, R.N. et al. (1995). Effect of Olsalazine on sodium-dependent bile acid transport in rat ileum. *Dig. Dis. Sci.* **40**:943–8.

Duncan, A., Cameron, A., Stewart, M.J. & Russell, R.I. (1991). Diagnosis of the abuse of magnesium and stimulant laxatives. *Ann. Clin. Biochem.* **28**:568–73.

Editorial (1990). Elderly people: Their medicines and their doctors. *Drugs Ther. Bull.* **28**:77–9.

Everhart, J.E., Go, V.L., Johannes, R.S., Fitzsimmons, S.C., Roth, H.P. & White, L.R. (1989). A longitudinal survey of self-reported bowel habits in the United States. *Dig. Dis. Sci.* **34**:1153–62.

Fortson, W.C. & Tedesco, F.J. (1984). Drug induced colitis: a review. *Am. J. Gastroenterol.* **79**:878–83.

Fromm, H., Tunuguntla, A.K., Malavolti, M., Sherman, C. & Ceryak, S. (1987). Absence of significant role of bile salts in diarrhoea of a heterogeneous group of postcholecystectomy patients. *Dig. Dis. Sci.* **32**:33–44.

Gurwitz, J.H., Noonan, J.P. & Soumerai, S.B. (1992). Reducing the use of H_2 receptor antagonists in the long term care setting. *J. Am. Geriatr. Soc.* **40**:359–64.

Hamilton, I., O'Connor, H.J., Wood, N.C., Bradbury, I. & Axon, A.T. (1986). Healing and recurrence of duodenal ulcer after treatment with tripotassium dicitrate bismuthate (TDB) tablets or cimetidine. *Gut* **27**:106–10.

Hurley, S.F., McNeil, J.J., Jolley, D.J. & Harvey, R. (1992). Linking prescription and patient-identifying data: a pilot study. *Med. J. Aust.* **156**:383–6.

Jackson, C.W., Haboubi, N.Y., Whorwell, P.J. & Schofield, P.F. (1986). Gold induced enterocolitis. *Gut* **27**:452–56.

Jarner, D. & Nielsen, M.A. (1983). Auranofin (SK+F39162) induced enterocolitis in rheumatoid arthritis. A case report. *Scand. J. Rheumatol.* **12**:254–6.

Kotzan, L., Carroll, N.V. & Kotzan, J.A. (1989). Influence of age, sex and race on prescription drug use among Georgia Medicaid recipients. *Am. J. Hosp. Pharm.* **46**:287–90.

Krejs, G.J. & Fordtran, J.S. (1985). Diarrhoea. In *Gastrointestinal Disease: Pathophysiology, Diagnosis, Management*, ed. M.H. Sleisenger & J.S. Fordtran, pp. 257–80. Philadelphia: Saunders.

Kruse, W., Rampmaier, J., Frauenrath-Volkers, C. et al. (1991). Drug prescribing patterns in old age. A study of the impact of hospitalization on drug prescriptions and follow-up survey in patients 75 years old and older. *Eur. J. Clin. Pharmacol.* **41**:441–7.

O'Brien, J., Thompson, D.G., Burnham, W.R. & Walker, E. (1986). Beta blocking drugs accelerate the passage of carbohydrate to the colon. *Gut* **27**:629.

Papadopoulos, C., Kalantzis, N., Rekoumis, G. & Kanaghinis, T. (1985). A comparative trial of 400 mg cimetidine twice daily and 1000 mg daily in the short-term treatment of duodenal ulceration. *Curr. Med. Res. Opin.* **9**:511–15.

Peterson, G.M., Mirkazemi, S., Friesen, W.T., Roberts, D. & Galloway, J.G. (1990). Diuretic use in institutionalized elderly Australians. *Aust. J. Hosp. Pharm.* **20**:302–4.

Phillips, S., Donaldson, L., Geisler, K., Pera, A. & Kochar, R. (1995). Stool composition in factitial diarrhea: a 6–year experience with stool analysis. *Ann. Intern. Med.* **123**:97–100.

Pokorra, M.D., Tett, S.E. & Higgins, G. (1991). NSAID use in a sample of elderly hospitalised patients. *Aust. J. Hosp. Pharm.* **21**:371–5.

Ratnaike, R.N. (1990). Diarrhoea in the elderly: epidemiological and aetiological factors. *J. Gastroenterol. Hepatol.* 5:449–58.

Ravdin, J.I. & Guerrant, R.L. (1983). Infectious diarrhoea in the elderly. *Geriatrics* 38:95–7, 99–101.

Simon, G.L. & Gorbach, S.L. (1986). The human intestinal microflora. *Dig. Dis. Sci.* 31:147S-62S.

Stewart, R.B., Moore, M.T., May, F.E., Marks, R.G. & Hale, W.E. (1991). Changing patterns of therapeutic agents in the elderly – a ten year overview. *Age Ageing* 20:182–8.

Thorens, J., Froehlich, F., Schwizer, W. et al. (1996). Bacterial overgrowth during treatment with omeprazole compared with cimetidine: a prospective randomised double blind study. *Gut* 39:54–9.

Walker, K.J., Gilliland, S.S., Vance-Bryan, K. et al. (1993) *Clostridium difficile* colonization in residents of long-term care facilities: prevalence and risk factors. *J. Am. Geriatr. Soc.* 41:940–6.

Wildeman, R.A. (1987). Focus on misoprostol: review of worldwide safety data. *Clin. Invest. Med.* 10:243–5.

8   Aetiology of infectious diarrhoea

Ranjit N. Ratnaike and David F.M. Looke

BACTERIA

Enteric infections are a major cause of acute diarrhoea in the elderly, due to diminished systemic and local gastrointestinal defences (see Chapters 1 and 2).Diarrhoea due to the ingestion of a pathogen is not invariable and depends on the number of organisms ingested (inoculum), their virulence and the efficiency of the host's defences. Other factors which predispose to diarrhoea in the elderly include current illnesses, poor personal and domestic hygiene as a result of mental and physical infirmities, and environmental constraints such as inadequate facilities for food preparation and preservation.

The elderly in institutions are at risk from common-source outbreaks of diarrhoea such as food poisoning and person to person transmission of enteric pathogens. In the elderly, nosocomial infections are common and pathogens frequently identified are *Clostridium difficile* and *Salmonella* sp. In a study on diarrhoea in the elderly from Britain, *Campylobacter jejuni* and nontyphoidal *Salmonella* and *Shigella* sp. were the most common organisms isolated.

The mechanisms by which bacteria cause diarrhoea are discussed elsewhere (see Chapter 3). Briefly, diarrhoea occurs either by the elaboration of a toxin which may act as a secretagogue (secretory agent) or as a cytotoxin, or by mucosal invasion, or a combination of these factors. Toxin can be preformed in food before ingestion or can be elaborated by the organism once established in the gastrointestinal tract.

Secretagogue production

An enterotoxin is traditionally accepted as an agent which causes secretion of water and electrolytes from the small intestine. The enterotoxins elaborated by the bacteria listed below, act as secretagogues on the epithelial cells of the small intestine.

Pre-formed toxin

- *Staphylococcus aureus*
- *Bacillus cereus*
- *Clostridium perfringens*

Toxin produced in situ

- *Vibrio cholerae*
- *Vibrio parahaemolyticus*
- Enterotoxigenic *E. coli* (ETEC)
- *Yersinia enterocolitica*
- *Aeromonas* sp.

Diarrhoea is mediated through elevations in the intracellular concentration of cyclic AMP or, less commonly, cyclic GMP (see Chapter 3). In essence, the toxin acts as a secretagogue and converts the function of the enterocyte from one of normal net absorption to net secretion. In secretory diarrhoea the bowel actions are voluminous and watery. Nausea and vomiting with cramping periumbilical abdominal pain is present to a variable extent. Cell damage does not occur and blood in the faeces is not a feature. Cholera toxin has acted as the most useful model for research on secretory toxins; however, many other organisms such as enterotoxigenic *E. coli* elaborate similar toxins.

Cytotoxin production

Cytotoxins cause cell injury and death. The bacteria which elaborate a cytotoxin are:

- *Shigella* sp.
  Shigella dysenteriae 1
  Shigella sonnei (some strains)
  Shigella flexneri (some strains)
- *Clostridium difficile*
- Enterohaemorrhagic *E. coli* (EHEC)
- *Campylobacter jejuni.*

Although complete evidence is still lacking, *C. jejuni* probably acts through cytotoxin production. The site of action of bacterial cytotoxins is usually in the ileum with frequent extension of infection to the colon.

Mucosal invasion

Bacterial invasion of epithelial cells is another major mechanism by which bacteria cause diarrhoea. These pathogens, listed below, predominantly affect the colon, although the lower small intestine is frequently involved:

- Enteroinvasive *E. coli* (EIEC)
- *Salmonella* sp.
- *Shigella* sp.
- *Campylobacter jejuni*
- *Yersinia enterocolitica*
- *Vibrio parahaemolyticus.*

Once the pathogen invades the cell, intracellular division and spread to adjacent cells occur. Cell death is invariably due to intracellular toxin production. A micro-ulcer or micro-abscess is formed when the dead cells are shed and an extensive inflammatory reaction in the lamina propria takes place.

The diarrhoeal stool consists of an inflammatory exudate, sloughed cells and cell debris, copious mucus from goblet cells, pus and blood. Dysentery is a term which refers to diarrhoea with blood and mucus and implies severe colonic infection. The bowel actions are frequent, of small volume with pus, mucus and often blood. Tenesmus, urgency, cramping and infraumbilical abdominal pain are prominent features. Constitutional symptoms such as pyrexia may be present. Faecal leuco-cytes are an important feature.

Many bacteria which cause diarrhoea have common features in regard to their mechanism of action, site of action and extra-intestinal manifestations. Patients with the HLA-B27 haplotype who are infected with *Shigella* sp., *Campylobacter jejuni* and *Yersinia enterocolitica* are predisposed to Reiter's syndrome.

Bacteria which produce secretagogues act on the small intestine, and those that elaborate cytotoxins and are invasive affect both the small and large intestine although the preferred site of infection is the ileum

Acute diarrhoea

Food-borne illness and food poisoning

The term food-borne illness, through recent frequent usage, includes the term food poisoning. Strictly, food poisoning implies the presence of a toxin in food, elab-orated by a pathogen. The symptoms are due to the toxin and not the pathogen. Food-borne illness requires the presence of the pathogen for the symptoms to occur. A food-borne disease outbreak is considered to have occurred if the follow-ing criteria are met:

(1)   two or more people experience the same symptoms, usually referable to the gas-trointestinal tract, after the consumption of the same dietary item

(2)   the dietary item is implicated as the common source by epidemiological investiga-tion.

Food poisoning is diagnosed when nausea, vomiting and diarrhoea occur after two to three persons have consumed the same food or beverage contaminated by a pre-formed toxin elaborated by a pathogen. The incubation period is short and the onset of symptoms is abrupt. The bacteria commonly implicated in food poisoning are:

- *Staphylococcus aureus*
- *Bacillus cereus*
- *Clostridium perfringens*
- *Vibrio parahaemolyticus.*

Viruses such as the Norwalk agent can produce an identical clinical picture.

Staphylococcus aureus

Profuse nausea, vomiting and diarrhoea one to six hours after a meal suggests ingestion of the preformed toxin elaborated by *S. aureus*. The vomiting is severe and metabolic alkalosis may occur. The symptoms resolve in about eight hours. Neurological symptoms such as numbness, tingling and vertigo may occur infrequently. A food handler with a pustule or paronychia, is a frequent source of food contamination. Growth of the organism in food is encouraged by inadequate refrigeration. Foods high in protein, sugar and salt, such as custards, cottage cheese and canned meat, are common sources of infection. The toxins can be heat stable or labile and therefore may not be inactivated by cooking. The food shows no evidence of the organism's activity and therefore appears normal, although the toxin is present. Since the symptoms are due to the toxin already elaborated in the food, antibiotics are irrelevant in the management. Treatment should be directed to prevent dehydration. Spontaneous recovery is the rule.

Bacillus cereus

B. cereus, a spore-forming organism, produces two symptom complexes. The first (the emetic illness) is of rapid onset and short duration, similar to that due to *S. aureus*, and is often associated with eating inadequately reheated fried rice. The temperature reached during 'flash frying' to reheat cold rice is insufficient to destroy the relatively heat-stable toxin. *B. cereus* is present in soil and contaminates uncooked rice: the process of cooking rice does not destroy the spores of the organism and when cooked rice is left to cool at room temperature the spores germinate and produce toxin. It is therefore important that cooked rice is refrigerated as soon as possible. The second symptom complex, in which abdominal pain and diarrhoea rather than vomiting predominate, is of longer onset and duration, and mimics infection due to *Clostridium perfringens* type A.

Clostridium perfringens

The toxin elaborated by *C. perfringens* type A is a component of the spore produced by the organism. The toxin may be preformed in food or elaborated by the organism within the small intestine. The vehicle of infection is usually a meat or poultry dish that was cooked, allowed to cool at room temperature (enabling the organism to multiply in the anaerobic conditions present and form more spores), and served a day or two later. The incubation period is 6 to 12 hours and the duration of illness about one day. The prominent symptoms are cramping abdominal pain and diarrhoea. Vomiting is infrequent. Constitutional symptoms are absent.

The toxin affects the lower small intestine and the occurrence of mucosal damage, malabsorption and protein loss have implications in elderly patients, many of whom are undernourished.

Although *C. perfringens* rarely causes antibiotic-associated diarrhoea, such an outbreak of diarrhoea has been reported in a geriatric unit. An enterocolitis similar to that due to *C. difficile* is reported, although pseudomembrane formation is not a feature. The treatment is with metronidazole.

In Papua New Guinea, eating undercooked pork together with sweet potato causes a necrotizing enterocolitis called 'pig-bel', due to *C. perfringens* type C.

Vibrio parahaemolyticus

V. parahaemolyticus is a form of food poisoning from contaminated seafood, particularly shellfish eaten raw or inadequately cooked. Outbreaks have occurred in Japan, USA, and Australia, although sporadic cases are the norm. The organism elaborates an enterotoxin which acts on the small intestine. The predominant symptom is watery diarrhoea together with abdominal cramps, nausea and vomiting, headache, fever and chills which usually resolve within three days. Less commonly, a dysenteric form of illness may occur. The diagnosis is established on stool culture. The treatment is symptomatic and the illness resolves in about a day.

Vibrio cholerae

The toxin of *V. cholerae* is a powerful secretagogue which causes severe watery diarrhoea associated with dehydration and substantial electrolyte depletion. Contaminated drinking water, containing large numbers of the organism, is the most common source of infection in outbreaks. An outbreak of cholera occurred in Peru in 1991 and has spread to seven other South American countries. The organism is an unlikely cause of diarrhoea in the developed world, although sporadic cases occur. In the clinical setting of voluminous, diarrhoeal stools which resemble 'rice water' the probability of cholera should be considered, especially if the patient is a traveller from an endemic area. Cholera is a rare cause of traveller's diarrhoea. A new strain of *V. cholerae* 'non-01 type' has arisen in India and is expected to spread slowly around the world.

Antibiotic therapy with tetracycline rapidly resolves the illness. Substantial fluid and electrolyte replacement are an essential part of management.

Salmonella infections

In the elderly the increase in the incidence, morbidity and mortality from *Salmonella* infections is well established. The genus *Salmonella* consists of one species and 2200 serotypes, which infect humans, animals and insects. Salmonellosis refers to the entire disease spectrum due to infection with *Salmonella*. The diagnosis is established by demonstrating the presence of the organism in stools or blood.

There are four major disease entities which may overlap. Each is due predominantly to a particular serotype of *Salmonella*:

- gastroenteritis most often due to *S. typhimurium*, and to strains such as *S. enteritidis*, *S. newport* or *S. anatum*
- enteric fever due to *S. typhi*, *S. paratyphi*, *S. schottmuelleri*, *S. hirschfeldi*
- extraintestinal infections following bacteraemia
- the asymptomatic carrier state (due to *S. typhi*).

Nontyphoidal *Salmonella*

Illness due to nontyphoidal *Salmonella* is a zoonosis, most commonly *S. typhimurium*, and is among the best documented and most common causes of diarrhoea in the western world. It is usually food-borne. The most common sources of infection are poultry and eggs. Inflammatory bowel disease is no longer considered a risk factor. In the elderly many factors increase the risk of infection with *Salmonella*:

- decrease in gastric acidity associated with aging and other factors discussed in Chapter 1
- the ingestion of the organism with agents that reduce gastric acidity, such as milk and milk products or therapeutic agents such as H_2 antagonists or proton pump inhibitors
- concurrent treatment with antibiotics; patients on antibiotics to which *Salmonella* are resistant are more susceptible to infection due to suppression of the protective normal bacterial flora of the colon
- malignancy
- states of decreased immunity.

When infection occurs, *Salmonella* adhere to and damage the microvilli of the epithelial cells in the terminal ileum by a toxin, and enter the cell. Here the organisms divide and enter the submucosa and are confined to the Peyer's patches. In patients with food-borne salmonellosis the illness is limited to the gastrointestinal tract.

The incubation period is 10 to 72 hours with an abrupt onset of diarrhoea, nausea, vomiting, abdominal pain and fever. The duration of illness lasts from one to four days and is usually self-limiting. The infection may spread to the colon and cause colitis.

In the elderly, especially those at risk, bacteraemia is a serious complication. It has been recommended that all elderly patients be treated with an antibiotic such as ciprofloxacin.

Typhoid fever

Enteric fever is a term of some antiquity which includes typhoid fever due to infection with *S. typhi* and paratyphoid fever due to *S. paratyphi A*, *S. schottmuelleri* or *S. hirschfeldi*. Typhoid fever is an acute, severe systemic illness characterized by fever and bacteraemia, abdominal pain and tenderness, hepatosplenomegaly, and rose spots, salmon-coloured maculopapular lesions, a characteristic rash which occurs during the second week.

In typhoid fever the bacteria are not confined to the Peyer's patches but spread to the mesenteric lymph nodes and then to the portal circulation. The organism proliferates within mononuclear phagocytic cells in the liver, spleen and lymph nodes and enters the blood stream to give rise to a second more intense wave of bacteraemia. The patient is febrile, the pulse rate is slow in comparison to the fever (relative bradycardia), the abdomen feels 'doughy' and loops of small intestine may be easily palpable.

Initially, constipation is followed by diarrhoea described as pea soup in consistency in about half the patients. The diarrhoeal component of the illness has been underestimated and recent reports from many countries emphasize the extent of the problem. The severity of diarrhoea in individual patients is reported to range from 3 to 30 stools per day.

Enterocolitis is a feature of variable severity. Toxic dilatation of the colon, severe haemorrhage and bowel perforation may occur. On sigmoidoscopy, in severe cases, hyperaemia, contact bleeding, granularity, friability and ulceration of the colonic mucosa are seen and are indistinguishable from ulcerative colitis.

Ciprofloxacin, chloramphenicol, ampicillin or sulfatrimethoprim are effective in the treatment of typhoid fever. Care must be taken in selecting an antimicrobial if the illness is acquired in a country where multi-drug-resistant disease exists. A quinolone would be the choice in this circumstance. Both live attenuated, killed and subunit vaccines exist for *S. typhi*. All have about 70 per cent efficacy and are recommended before travel to areas where the disease is endemic.

Extraintestinal complications

In the elderly, serious extraintestinal complications may result from enteric fever, or from the rare occurrence of bacteraemia as a complication of nontyphoidal food-borne illness. Among the nontyphoidal serotypes of *Salmonella* the risk of bacteraemia is greatest with *S. cholerasuis*. The sites of infection relevant to the elderly (especially endothelial surfaces of the cardiovascular system) are:

- cardiac prostheses
- damaged cardiovascular endothelial surfaces
- infrarenal atherosclerotic aortic aneurysms
- mural thrombi
- necrotic tumours
- haematomas
- skeletal prostheses
- axial and peripheral joints
- long bones.

Joints commonly involved in suppurative arthritis are the knee, shoulder, hip and sacroiliac joints. Aseptic polyarthritis also occurs. Extraintestinal complications in the elderly may require extensive investigations to establish the extent of infection before treatment. The therapy may involve surgical intervention together with appropriate parenteral antibiotics.

Chronic asymptomatic carriers

About 3 per cent of adults infected with *S. typhi* continue to harbour the organism and become chronic asymptomatic carriers. A chronic carrier is defined as a person who excretes *Salmonella* for 12 months or more. The carrier state is more common among the elderly, especially females, and those with biliary tract disease. Urinary tract carriage of the organism occurs with an obstructive uropathy or schistosomiasis. Chronic asymptomatic carriers should be monitored for one year and, if excretion of the organism persists, should be treated with a four- to six-week course of ciprofloxacin or amoxycillin. If this therapy fails, a cholecystectomy under antibiotic cover, and ampicillin or amoxycillin for two weeks, resolves the problem in 90 per cent of cases.

Escherichia coli

Increasing numbers of strains of *E. coli* that cause diarrhoea are being described, resulting in an ever changing taxonomic status. Some 'types' of *E. coli* which cause diarrhoea are:

- enterotoxigenic *E. coli* (ETEC)
- enteropathogenic *E. coli* (EPEC)
- enteroadhesive *E. coli* (EAEC)
- enteroinvasive *E. coli* (EIEC)
- enterohaemorrhagic *E. coli* (EHEC)

Certain strains of *E.coli* generally accord with a pathogenic type; e.g. *E.coli* 0157:H7 is the major strain of enterohaemorrhagic *E.coli* (EHEC). Enterotoxigenic *E. coli* (ETEC), enteropathogenic *E. coli* (EPEC) and enteroadhesive *E. coli* (EAEC)infect the small intestine to cause watery diarrhoea. Infections of the colon occur with enteroinvasive *E. coli* (EIEC) and enterohaemorrhagic *E. coli* (EHEC).

Enterotoxigenic *E. coli* (ETEC)

Infection occurs by ingestion of contaminated food or water. Enterotoxigenic *E. coli* (ETEC) is the most common cause of traveller's diarrhoea and is associated primarily with diarrhoea in young children in the developing world. The major symptom is profuse watery diarrhoea due to the heat-stable, cholera-like toxin. The disease is usually self-limiting, although treatment with antibiotics, such as sulfatrimethoprim or a quinolone, significantly shortens the duration of illness.

Enteropathogenic *E. coli* (EPEC)

This organism causes cell damage by first adhering to the microvilli of the epithelial cell mediated by an adherence factor and then by the liberation of a cytotoxin. Characteristically, the diarrhoea is watery. The extent to which this pathogen causes diarrhoea in the elderly is not yet known.

Enteroadhesive *E. coli* (EAEC)

Enteroadhesive *E. coli* (EAEC) also damages the epithelial cell through adherence and is a less common cause of traveller's diarrhoea.

Enteroinvasive *E. coli* (EIEC)

Enteroinvasive *E. coli* (EIEC), although an infrequent cause of diarrhoea, is implicated in food-borne infectious diarrhoea and traveller's diarrhoea. This invasive pathogen multiplies within the epithelial cells of the distal ileum and the colon. The clinical picture is of diarrhoea with blood and mucus, abdominal pain, tenesmus and systemic symptoms of fever and myalgia, indistinguishable from *Salmonella* or *Campylobacter* clinically. Treatment is with sulfatrimethoprim or norfloxacin.

Enterohaemorrhagic *E. coli* (EHEC)

The natural reservoir of this organism is the gastrointestinal tract of animals. Contaminated animal products, especially inadequately cooked ground beef in fast foods such as hamburgers, meat pies and tacos, are the most common source of infection.

E. coli 0157:H7 is the recently identified predominant serotype of enterohaemorrhagic *E. coli* and is responsible for severe haemorrhagic colitis due to two toxins, verotoxin I and verotoxin II. The organism does not invade the colonic mucosa.

The most vulnerable are the elderly and the very young. An outbreak in a nursing home in Canada highlighted the high mortality associated with this entity. The initial symptoms are those of watery diarrhoea and abdominal pain. Bloody diarrhoea and abdominal cramps may follow some days later. Fever is not a part of the illness. The organism may also cause an asymptomatic infection or a mild nonbloody diarrhoea. The haemolytic uraemic syndrome and thrombotic thrombocytopenic purpura are major life-threatening complications. At present, the role of antibiotic therapy is unclear.

Campylobacter jejuni

The incidence of infections due to this zoonotic pathogen is increasing; 50 to 70 per cent of infections with *C. jejuni* are associated with poultry. Important nonpoultry sources of infection are contaminated milk and milk products. The transmission of *Campylobacter* to humans from household pets, such as dogs and cats, with diarrhoea is reported. The exact mechanism of action of *C. jejuni* on the gut epithelium is uncertain, although cytotoxin production is most likely.

In the majority of healthy persons, diarrhoea is invariably self-limiting and settles within seven days. The disease spectrum ranges from small intestinal involvement with mild diarrhoea and cramping abdominal pain, to fulminating colitis associated with fatalities. The colonic lesions are similar to Crohn's disease and ulcerative colitis. Complications include toxic megacolon, carditis, arthritis, pneumonia, infections of the urinary tract and the Guillain–Barre syndrome.

Treatment is warranted in elderly patients with prolonged bloody diarrhoea and pyrexia, severe concomitant illnesses, and those who are debilitated. The drug of choice at present is erythromycin as quinolone resistance is rapidly emerging.

Shigella sp.

Humans are the only reservoirs of *Shigella*. The organism is highly contagious. Infection can occur with as small an inoculum as 10^2 organisms. The four sero groups are *S. sonnei*, common in the developing world, *S.dysenteriae 1*, *S. flexneri* and *S. boydii*. The most virulent of the organisms, *S. dysenteriae 1*, is associated with a protein-losing enteropathy.

The initial symptoms of nausea and vomiting, and watery diarrhoea, are due to enterotoxin liberation and absorption in the small intestine during the passage of the organism to the colon. If the infection is limited to the small intestine these symptoms resolve in less than a week. In colonic infections the organism penetrates the mucosa and liberates a cytotoxin which causes cell death. Mucosal inflammation, ulceration and crypt abscesses occur, leading to dysentery.

Infection with *Shigella* is relevant to the elderly on many counts. In a study on shigellosis in Israel over a ten-year period, 32 of 116 patients were over 70 years of age and the most frequent extragastrointestinal symptom was confusion. The protein-losing enteropathy has implications in undernourished or malnourished patients. Shiga toxin can also cause haemolytic uraemic syndrome (HUS) as it is similar in action to the verotoxin produced by enterohaemorrhagic *E. coli* (EHEC). The treatment is with sulfatrimethoprim or a quinolone.

Clostridium difficile

C. difficile is a frequent cause of diarrhoea in the elderly. The institutionalized elderly, patients on long-term antibiotic therapy, and those on chemotherapy for malignancy, are particularly susceptible. After oral or parenteral antibiotic administration an altered colonic environment is created, depleted of bacteria proactive to the host. This facilitates infection with *C. difficile* which then produces a number of toxins. The precise pathogenic mechanisms are still being debated.

The antibiotics most frequently associated with *C. difficile*-associated colitis are clindamycin, cephalosporins and ampicillin. Virtually all antibiotics have been implicated including vancomycin and metronidazole which, paradoxically, are the drugs used for the treatment of *C.difficile*-associated colitis. Amoxycillin and ampicillin are cited most often as the cause of *C. difficile* infection because of their widespread use. There is no causal relationship between the type of antibiotic or the dose, nor with the onset or the duration and severity of diarrhoea. The onset of diarrhoea even a month after a course of antibiotics does not discount infection due to *C. difficile.*

The organism elaborates two toxins, a hypersecretory toxin A and a cytopathic toxin B. Infection with *C. difficile* and pseudomembraneous colitis are closely associated but are not synonymous. The consequences of infection with *C. difficile* vary from mild watery diarrhoea in the absence of colitis, through colitis with no pseudomembrane formation, to 'true' pseudomembraneous colitis.

The pseudomembrane is a raised, discrete, creamy-yellow plaque about 2 cm in diameter and composed of a layer of fibrin, mucin, inflammatory cells, dead epithelial cells and goblet cells. The pseudomembrane may be present only in the proximal colon and not in the rectum.

A protein-losing enteropathy associated with *C. difficile* infection was diagnosed in the majority of a group of 38 patients over the age of 60 years. In 12 patients in this group colonized with *C. difficile* but with neither diarrhoea nor pseudomembrane formation, protein loss was detected in six patients. This finding may contribute to undernutrition in asymptomatic elderly patients. Rare complications are toxic megacolon and colonic perforation.

The diagnosis is usually confirmed by the demonstration of cytotoxin in the faeces. Culture of the organism alone is a poor diagnostic indication as it may be present in asymptomatic individuals.

In the majority of cases, antibiotic treatment is not necessary and cessation of antibiotics is all that is required. In resistant cases, oral metronidazole, vancomycin or bacitracin is used. In a British study, vancomycin rather than metronidazole was the preferred drug due to greater efficacy and fewer side effects. Vancomycin is expensive and, to avoid the development of widespread resistance, it is preferable to restrict its use to severe diarrhoea unresponsive to metronidazole or bacitracin.

Recurrences are documented in about one third of patients treated with vancomycin and, therefore, the convalescence of elderly patients should be monitored after treatment. When a relapse occurs, in addition to prolonged therapy with vancomycin for 14 days, measures to improve personal hygiene, such as frequent hand washing especially after using the toilet and before meals and, in a hospital or nursing home setting, more rigorous ward cleaning, should be promoted. The spores of *C. difficile* survive for up to five months and have been isolated from sources such as bedding and bedpans. There are some preliminary reports that co-treatment with oral yeast preparations improves outcome and prevents relapse.

Yersinia enterocolitica

In an Australian study on adult diarrhoea in the community *Y. enterocolitica* was the third most common bacterial pathogen identified, after *C. jejuni* and nontyphoidal *Salmonella*.

Infected food, particularly pork, is the most common source of infection although the organism may be present in natural water sources. Epidemics have been reported following the ingestion of chocolate milk, pasteurized milk, ice cream, tofu (a soya bean preparation), and bean sprouts. Unlike other pathogens the organism can continue to grow at 4°C, the temperature of a refrigerator. As with *Campylobacter jejuni*, *Y. enterocolitica* has been isolated from domestic pets and farm animals and is generally regarded as a zoonotic pathogen.

The major symptoms are similar to *Campylobacter* infections. In some patients right lower quadrant pain and fever may mimic appendicitis. In the elderly, septicaemia is an uncommon but serious complication. Extraintestinal multisystem infection and recurrences are reported in a proportion of patients. A rash and arthralgia occur in individuals with the HLA-B27 haplotype. Terminal ileal involvement mimics Crohn's disease.

Infection with *Y. enterocolitica* is self-limiting in the healthy subject. In the elderly person at risk, or if complications of extraintestinal infection occur, the drugs of choice are aminoglycosides or quinolones.

Aeromonas species

Infection with *Aeromonas* spp. may present as a dysentery-like syndrome or mimic inflammatory bowel disease. A feature of interest is prolonged infection which leads to chronic diarrhoea. The source of infection is usually through contaminated water.

Chronic diarrhoea

Mycobacterium tuberculosis

Intestinal tuberculosis is a rarity in developed countries. This condition should be considered as a cause of chronic diarrhoea particularly in migrants from countries where tuberculosis is prevalent. In addition to diarrhoea, significant weight loss, fever and night sweats, abdominal pain, and a 'doughy' feeling on abdominal palpation due to oedematous intestines, are prominent clinical features.

The lesion is an annular or oval ulcer usually in the ileum and the caecum. The complications include small intestinal narrowing, stricture formation, fistulas and bacterial overgrowth. The treatment consists of antituberculous therapy as for pulmonary tuberculosis.

PARASITES

The parasitic causes of diarrhoea are not confined to the developing world. In the West the importance of many of these pathogens, including *Cryptosporidium*, in the aetiology of diarrhoea has been highlighted since the advent of AIDS.

Parasitic infection of the gastrointestinal tract does not inevitably lead to diarrhoea as many individuals are asymptomatic carriers. Diarrhoea is the outcome between the defences of the host and the virulence of the parasite. In good health, a greater parasitic load (inoculum) is required to cause disease, while in the extremes of age due to host vulnerability a smaller inoculum suffices. For the reasons discussed in Chapters 1 and 2, the elderly patient is vulnerable to infection. Parasitic infection of the gastrointestinal tract and diarrhoea are not infrequent sequelae of immunosuppression due to drug therapy or disease.

In contrast to acute diarrhoea due to a viral or bacterial aetiology, the temporal profile of diarrhoea due to parasites is different: chronicity is more likely.

In this chapter, parasites which rarely cause an infection in healthy subjects are discussed because of their importance in the aetiology of diarrhoea in the immunosuppressed. Other intestinal parasites, although pathogenic, are not discussed as diarrhoea is not a significant feature of the illness.

The parasites which are associated with diarrhoea are:

Protozoa

- *Giardia lamblia*
- *Entamoeba histolytica*
- *Cryptosporidium*
- *Isospora belli*
- *Microsporidia*
- *Sarcocystis hominis*
- *Balantidium coli*
- *Blastocystis hominis*

Nematodes (round worms)

- *Strongyloides stercoralis*
- *Trichuris trichiura*

- *Capillaria philippinensis*
- *Trichinella spiralis.*

Trematodes (flukes)

- *Schistosoma mansoni*
- *Schistosoma japonicum.*

The majority of the diarrhoea-causing organisms are protozoans. Class sporozoa is one of the four classes of the phylum protozoa.

Infection is by cysts (or oocysts in sporozoa) through the faeco-oral route, by person-to-person contact and contaminated food and water. The faeco-oral route is the most frequent pathway of entry. Less commonly, the faeco-oral route may be bypassed, avoiding the nonimmunological and immunological gastrointestinal defences. The parasite may enter per rectum through enemas for colonic irrigation to 'cleanse the bowel' (a service offered by some nonallopathic health practitioners), or through inadequately reprocessed surgical instruments. The cysts of protozoa are capable of prolonged survival in the soil and are resistant to drying. In the elderly, decreased gastric acid concentrations enable more cysts to survive the gastric acid barrier.

The spread of infective cysts from asymptomatic carriers and patients with diarrhoea occurs when the elderly are in close contact and share facilities, as in nursing homes and psychogeriatric wards. In such environments a patient with infective diarrhoea, faecal incontinence and poor personal hygiene due to dementia, poses a great risk to others.

Enteric parasites cause diarrhoea through diverse mechanisms. Parasiticinfection of the small intestine may lead to malabsorption and diarrhoea, and colonic infections may lead to dysentery. In some instances, as with *Giardia lamblia*, diarrhoea occurs due to mucosal damage of the small bowel. The pathogenesis of abnormal villous architecture is speculative; perhaps a toxin is responsible. Cryptosporidium invades the enterocyte, but does not enter the cytoplasm, occupying an extracytoplasmic position beneath the apical membrane. The mechanism of diarrhoea is possibly by a secretagogue elaborated by *Cryptosporidium*; the bowel actions are voluminous and watery. *Entamoeba histolytica* invades and extensively damages the large intestinal epithelial cells, and diarrhoea is often bloodstained and purulent.

Host responses to infection vary with the site of infection and the extent of damage the parasite causes. *Strongyloides stercoralis*, a nematode worm, invades the mucosa of the small intestine and is associated with a high eosinophil response. Eosinophilia is not an inevitable consequence of parasitic infections but occurs as a result of mucosal invasion by the pathogen. Intestinal parasites which cause diarrhoea and eosinophilia are:

Protozoa

- *Isospora belli*
- *Sarcocystis hominis.*

Nematodes (round worms)

- *Strongyloides stercoralis*
- *Trichuris trichiura*
- *Trichinella spiralis.*

Trematodes (flukes)

- *Schistosoma mansoni*
- *Schistosoma japonicum.*

Protozoa

Giardia lamblia

In the Western world, *Giardia lamblia*, a flagellate protozoan, is the most common parasite to infect the small intestine. The majority who harbour this organism are asymptomatic. Although children are the major reservoir of disease, *G. lamblia* is a major cause of diarrhoea in the elderly who have travelled to areas of inadequate sanitation where the parasite is endemic or who are in contact with infected children. Infection is reported to occur by the ingestion of as few as ten cysts.

Outbreaks of diarrhoea have occurred amongst visitors to the snowfields of USA in Aspen and Boulder, Colorado; New Zealand; and to St. Petersburg (formerly Leningrad), Russia. Household pets such as dogs and cats act as a reservoir of infection. In a study from the south east of England, *Giardia* cysts were found in the faeces of 20 per cent of dogs and 35 per cent of cats, although none had diarrhoea. Many animal strains are not pathogenic for humans.

The symptoms occur about two weeks after infection and include abdominal discomfort, distension, flatulence and diarrhoea. The predominant symptom, diarrhoea, may occur acutely, intermittently, or be chronic due to malabsorption. Reinfection is frequent.

The morphology of the small intestine shows mucosal inflammation and varying degrees of villous atrophy. The mechanism of these changes is not established. Patients with chronic diarrhoea have been misdiagnosed as having irritable bowel syndrome or coeliac disease. Other factors, in addition to villous atrophy, which may account for malabsorption include bacterial overgrowth and subsequent bile salt deconjugation (see Chapter 9).

Giardiasis is diagnosed by the presence of cysts in faeces; or trophozoites and/or cysts in specimens of small intestinal mucosa or duodenal aspirates. The highest diagnostic yield is from examination of the mucosal biopsy. Examination of the stool for cysts, which are shed cyclically, is least rewarding, but most easily performed. Three separate stool examinations are required to maximize the yield from this test. Peripheral blood eosinophilia is not a feature, nor is the ESR elevated. The treatment of choice is with metronidazole or tinidazole. Quinacrine and furazolidone are second-line agents.

Entamoeba histolytica

Amoebiasis is a condition in which *Entamoeba histolytica* is harboured with or without clinical symptoms. There are many strains of *E. histolytica* and only some are pathogenic. Current routine laboratory techniques cannot differentiate between strains.

E. histolytica exists both in the cyst form and as a trophozoite; the latter is vulnerable to gastric acid and is unable to survive in an environment outside the colon. In the majority of individuals (85 to 95 per cent) the parasite is a harmless commensal of the large intestine. *E. histolytica* as a cause of chronic diarrhoea should be suspected in the elderly who are institutionalized or have visited the tropics, although a significant number of cases are diagnosed each year in the USA in the absence of a history of foreign travel. The organism has been found in up to 30 per cent of asymptomatic gay men. Animals are not an important source of infection.

Isolation and characterization of isoenzymes (zymodemes) from species of *Entamoeba histolytica* has identified nonpathogenic and pathogenic strains which explains the varied severity in infection, from asymptomatic carriage to disseminated, fatal disease.

The right colon is the common site of infection, followed by the rectum, the sigmoid colon, the appendix and the terminal ileum. Diarrhoea, associated with abdominal tenderness, may present as a few loose, bulky bowel actions per day or in severe cases as dysentery. In chronic amoebic dysentery, diarrhoea may alternate with constipation. Fulminant or necrotizing colitis, a rare complication, is associated with a 60 per cent mortality.

An uncommon initial presentation is the amoeboma, a localized granulomatous caecal lesion which may be mistaken for a colonic malignancy. The most common sites are the caecum (40 per cent) and rectosigmoid colon (20 per cent). Liver abscess is another complication, and usually involves the right lobe. These complications usually occur in the absence of diarrhoea.

Sigmoidoscopy may be normal since ulceration occurs predominantly in the caecum and ascending colon. For this reason, colonoscopy is the preferred investigation. The typical amoebic ulcers are shallow, 2 cm or more in diameter, with raised edges and a yellowish exudate. The mucosa between ulcers is normal. In the elderly, the colon is reported to become oedematous and friable and damage may occur during sigmoidoscopy.

The definitive diagnosis of amoebiasis is based on the detection of either trophozoites or cysts in fresh (within half an hour of passage) samples of faeces, or in exudates obtained during sigmoidoscopy or colonoscopy. Often, repeated examinations of stool specimens are necessary to establish a diagnosis. Serological tests are useful to establish a diagnosis of extraintestinal, tissue-invasive amoebiasis as in an amoebic liver abscess.

The treatment of choice in intestinal disease is metronidazole followed by diloxanide furoate. Asymptomatic carriers should also be treated with diloxanide furoate.

Amoebic dysentery has been frequently misdiagnosed as inflammatory bowel disease. A recent report from South Korea emphasizes the dangers of misdiagnosis and treatment with steroids, and delay in instituting antiamoebic therapy.

Coccidia

The genus *Cryptosporidium* and *Isospora* belong to the subclass Coccidia. The word coccidiosis is derived from the Greek, kokkos=berry, eidos=form, and osis=condition. Human coccidiosis is due to *Cryptosporidium parvum*, *Isospora belli*, *Microsporidia*, *Cyclospora cayetanensis* or, rarely, *Sarcocystis hominis* (formerly called *Isospora hominis*). These parasites may cause severe diarrhoea in association with HIV infections and other states of immunosuppression. The site of infection is the small intestinal epithelial cell.

Cryptosporidium parvum

In immunocompetent individuals, principally in children, Cryptosporidium causes a self-limited illness dominated by diarrhoea, with anorexia, nausea and vomiting, and sometimes a low grade fever. In those immunocompromised, the diarrhoea is severe and prolonged, accompanied by significant weight loss. The parasite is a well established cause of traveller's diarrhoea.

The small intestinal morphology shows varying degrees of villous atrophy, crypt hyperplasia and increased numbers of eosinophils and plasma cells in the lamina propria. *Cryptosporidium* may also damage the colonic mucosa. The diagnosis is usually made by detecting oocysts in the faeces by the use of modified acid-fast strains. Identification of the parasite in biopsy material is a more sensitive method, should the stools be negative. There are no antimicrobial agents that have been proven to be beneficial against *Cryptosporidium*, although anecdotal evidence supports the use of paromomycin. An immunofluorescence test to detect an antigen of the oocyst wall is now available.

It is possible that the diarrhoea is mediated by a secretagogue and the beneficial use of octreotide, a somatostatin analogue, supports this speculation.

Isospora belli

Most individuals who harbour this parasite are asymptomatic carriers. In others, particularly those immunocompromised, severe diarrhoea, abdominal cramps, nausea and vomiting with fever and headache may last for a few days to weeks. Malabsorption due to small intestinal mucosal damage leads to chronic diarrhoea. In the alimentary canal other areas of involvement are the oesophagus and colon.

The possibility of isosporiasis in an immunocompetent patient with obscure chronic diarrhoea must not be regarded as exotic. A patient with intermittent diarrhoea for 20 years due to *Isospora belli* has been described.

The diagnosis is made by examination of the faeces for oocysts, or duodenal juice, and a small bowel biopsy for the organism which may be seen in various developmental stages. *Isospora belli* is the only protozoan intestinal parasite to cause eosinophilia but the absence of eosinophilia does not negate the diagnosis. Eosinophilia occurs in about 50 per cent of patients. Sulfatrimethoprim is the treatment of choice for chronic diarrhoea.

Microsporidia

The microsporidia *Enterocytozoon bieneusi* and *Septata intestinalis*, are a well documented cause of chronic diarrhoea in HIV-infected individuals. They are diagnosed by examination of small bowel biopsy, duodenal aspirate or faeces specimen. Albendazole and octreotide have been useful in the treatment. Other microsporidian species have been identified less commonly in patients with AIDS.

Information on intestinal parasites which do not commonly cause diarrhoea in the western world is given in an appendix at the end of this chapter.

VIRUSES

During the past two decades, viruses have joined bacteria and parasites as important causes of diarrhoea in the elderly. Although virus-caused diarrhoea is usually seen in children, sporadic cases and epidemic outbreaks are seen in adults and the elderly.

Virus diarrhoea occurs as one of two main clinical scenarios. First, viruses such as Rotavirus and Calicivirus cause sporadic cases or epidemics in those with normal health and are acquired illnesses. Secondly, viruses may cause diarrhoea when a chronic carrier state is reactivated as a result of immunosuppression, for example Cytomegalovirus (CMV), or as part of a generalized viral infection such as human immunodeficiency virus (HIV) infection.

The viruses which cause human gastroenteritis can be grouped into five major categories: Rotavirus, 'enteric' adenovirus, Norwalk virus, Astrovirus and Calicivirus.

Rotavirus infection is classically seen in infants, but, frequent case reports in older people demonstrate that the illness is not restricted to the younger age group. Rotaviruses are members of the Reovirus family and are nonenveloped double-stranded RNA viruses. There are three major antigenic groups, known as group A, B and C with group A Rotaviruses causing the majority of disease.

Although a large proportion of Rotaviral infection is asymptomatic, disease usually occurs after an incubation period of one to three days. Symptoms are typically those of vomiting and watery diarrhoea and usually last from three to eight days, with vomiting being predominant for the first 36 hours. A history of contact with a young child with diarrhoea strengthens the diagnosis of an infection with Rotavirus. Viral shedding can continue for up to 21 days. The diagnosis is most often made by enzymeimmunoassay (EIA) of the stool for Rotavirus antigen.

Treatment is symptomatic with correction of dehydration being of paramount importance. The illness is nearly always self-limiting. Epidemics of Rotavirus infection have been reported in geriatric populations.

Enteric adenoviruses are noncultivatable strains of adenovirus which are categorized as serotypes 40 and 41. In contrast to the common strains of adenovirus which cause respiratory illness or conjunctivitis, enteric adenoviruses cause gastroenteritis with no respiratory symptoms. Disease follows an incubation of eight to ten days and is usually manifested by watery diarrhoea followed by one to two days of vomiting. Fever is not prominent and the illness lasts from five to twelve days.

The diagnosis is usually made by EIA of the stool, but further identification of the viruses is usually performed only by certain research groups. Nosocomial outbreaks have been reported.

Norwalk virus is the prototype of a group of noncultivatable viruses usually named after the city where they were isolated from patients who were part of an epidemic of vomiting illness. Although the virus cannot be cultivated it has been characterized as a nonenveloped single-stranded RNA virus. Genetic analysis reveals that it is a type of Calicivirus.

Norwalk virus or serologically related viruses cause up to 40 per cent of outbreaks of gastroenteritis in camps, cruise ships, families, nursing homes and hospital wards, or outbreaks that follow the ingestion of shellfish or contaminated water. Air-borne transmission may occur. Infection occurs in all age groups.

The incubation period is 12–48 hours and the predominant symptom is vomiting as well as watery diarrhoea. Because of the frequency of occurrence during winter, it has been called 'winter vomiting disease'. The illness lasts for one to two days only and is self-limiting, but the virus may be excreted for up to 48 hours after the cessation of symptoms. The diagnosis may be made by electron microscopic examination of the stools or vomitus; however, characterization of the agent is limited to a few reference laboratories. EIA of stool is a sensitive and specific test, but not yet widely available.

The Caliciviruses are less well understood as causes of diarrhoea. They are non-cultivatable, nonenveloped, single-stranded RNA viruses which infect a wide variety of animal species. The human strains either cause asymptomatic infection or gastroenteritis. The incubation period is 24–72 hours and the illness is generally mild with watery diarrhoea, abdominal cramps and vomiting. The symptoms are usually self-limited and last from one to three days. The diagnosis may be made by electron microscopy of stool specimens. Epidemics within nursing homes have been reported.

There have been at least five serotypes of human Astrovirus characterized. They are cultivatable, nonenveloped, single-stranded RNA viruses, similar to but distinct from Caliciviruses. Although Astrovirus infection is usually reported in children, reports of diarrhoea in all age groups have been made, and outbreaks in geriatric facilities have been reported.

The incubation period is probably three to four days and the clinical illness of diarrhoea and constitutional symptoms are mild. Vomiting is prominent. The illness is usually self-limiting and lasts from two to three days. The diagnosis can be made by electron microscopy of the stools, and recently an EIA test for viral antigens has been described, but is not yet widely available.

Viruses that do not cause gastroenteritis as their primary manifestation may cause diarrhoea as part of their symptom complex. This is usually in the circumstance of immunosuppression. Cytomegalovirus infection of the gastrointestinal tract (GIT) occurs with severe immunosuppression, as seen in the later stages of human immunodeficiency virus (HIV) infection or following organ transplantation. Reactivation of latent infection occurs and, as well as other organs being involved, the GIT may suffer significantly. Small bowel involvement leads to villous atrophy, malabsorption and chronic diarrhoea. A colitis may also develop with bloody diarrhoea and ulceration of the colon.

The diagnosis is made from biopsy where characteristic viral inclusions are seen in the nuclei of enterocytes, endothelial cells and fibroblasts. Treatment with Ganciclovir, Foscarnet or Cidofovir may achieve a measure of success. Diarrhoea commonly occurs in the latter stages of infection with the human immuno-deficiency virus (HIV). Although in the majority of cases it is caused by opportunistic infection such as *Cryptosporidium*, microsporidiosis, Cytomegalovirus (mentioned above), nontuberculous mycobacterial infection, Rotaviruses, Enteroviruses, *Entamoeba histolytica*, giardiasis and strongyloidiasis, or malignancy such as Kaposi's sarcoma or GIT lymphoma, diarrhoea may occur in the absence of any of the above.

An enteropathy caused by HIV infection has been described which causes watery diarrhoea, malabsorption and weight loss. This entity may prove to be an as yet diagnosed opportunistic infection. Therapy should be directed toward any pathogen isolated. Symptomatic treatment such as loperamide is helpful. The somatostatin analogue octreotide has proven useful in severe refractory cases. Maximal suppression of HIV with combination antiretroviral therapy, if successful, often results in significant reversal of symptoms, weight gain and improvement in well being. This is particularly so if the patient has not been previously treated.

APPENDIX
INFORMATION ON UNUSUAL PARASITES WHICH CAUSE DIARRHOEA

Protozoa

Sarcocystis hominis

Sarcocystis hominis infects the small intestine and produces symptoms similar to those caused by *Isospora belli*. The diagnosis is made by identifying oocysts in faeces or in duodenal fluid or biopsy.

Neither *Isospora belli* nor *Sarcocystis hominis* require a vector and the infective oocysts survive for long periods in the soil.

Treatment: Trimethoprim-sulfamethoxazole is used to treat *Isospora belli* and *Sarcocystis hominis*. In AIDS patients, more than one treatment course may be required or, in some instances, maintenance therapy will have to be instituted.

Balantidium coli

Balantidium coli is the largest protozoan which infects man. It is commonly found in pigs. Infection is through cysts. After excystation in the colon the trophozoite, like *E. histolytica*, invades the colon to cause ulceration, abscess formation, diarrhoea and rectal bleeding. In the absence of colonic invasion the patient is asymptomatic, or the clinical picture may be one of mild intermittent diarrhoea.

The diagnosis is established by the presence of the trophozoite or cysts in the stools. Treatment is with tetracycline.

Blastocystis hominis

This protozoan parasite is frequently isolated from stools, but its role in causing diarrhoea remains controversial, and it remains a diagnosis of exclusion. Metronidazole appears to have some benefit.

Nematodes (round worms)

Strongyloides stercoralis

The nematode *S. stercoralis* is an important intestinal parasite with a world wide distribution. Transmission of the pathogen occurs by the faecocutaneous route. Autoinfection and infection among inmates of institutions is common. In the upper small intestine the diminutive female, 2 mm in length, burrows into the mucosa and lays her eggs. The intestinal phase is characterized by diarrhoea alternating with constipation. The other clinical features are urticaria, abdominal pain and pruritus ani. Instances of intestinal obstruction, paralytic ileus and malabsorption are reported. A hyperinfection syndrome is well described in the context of immunosuppression with corticosteroids.

Small bowel changes of villous atrophy occur with varying severity.

Eosinophilia is a major finding and the eosinophil count may be as high as 20 000 cells per ml of blood. The diagnosis is made by finding larvae in faeces, duodenal fluid or in a biopsy of the small intestine. Serology may be helpful.

Treatment: Thiabendazole is often only partially effective and more than one treatment course may be required, particularly in the immunosuppressed. An alternative is Albendazole.

Trichuris trichiura

Trichuris trichiura is one of the most common nematodes which causes intestinal infections in humans. The adult worm is 30 to 50mm in length. The infection is acquired through ingestion of eggs from faeces in the soil. The eggs hatch in the small intestine and the larvae migrate to and mature in the large intestine.

Although asymptomatic infection is the norm, the symptoms may consist of abdominal pain, diarrhoea and dysentery. Rectal prolapse may occur with massive infection.

The diagnosis is made by identifying the eggs in faeces.

Treatment: Mebendazole

Capillaria philippinensis

C. philippinensis causes intestinal capillariasis, a rare disease first recognized in Luzon, Philippines. The organism, 2–4 mm in length, invades the small intestinal mucosa. The major manifestations are a severe protein-losing enteropathy and persistent watery diarrhoea. The diagnosis is established by the presence of ova in the faeces. The ova resemble those of *Tr. trichiura*, which may coexist.

Treatment: Mebendazole.

Trichinella spiralis

Trichinella spiralis is widely distributed in many parts of the world although trichinosis is an uncommon illness. Humans are incidental hosts who acquire the infection through eating undercooked meat, usually pork. The larvae are released in the stomach when the cyst wall is digested. Adulthood is reached in the wall of the small intestine. Larvae are then produced which migrate to, and encyst within, striated muscle.

Diarrhoea is an initial symptom. In one to two weeks other clinical features occur: fever, myositis and periorbital oedema. The small bowel biopsy shows features of villous atrophy and an inflammatory infiltrate of the lamina propria. Eosinophilia is a constant finding. The serum creatine kinase is elevated due to muscle involvement. The diagnosis is made clinically and confirmed by serology or rarely by muscle biopsy.

Treatment: Thiabendazole may be of some benefit but many authorities consider that no definite therapy is available.

Trematodes

Schistosoma mansoni and *Schistosoma japonicum*

Schistosomiasis due to infection with *S. mansoni* or *S. japonicum* is a rare cause of diarrhoea (with or without blood), but is more likely to present with haematuria. Chronic long-term infection may lead to massive hepatosplenomegaly with hepatic cirrhosis and portal hypertension. Eosinophilia is a feature. The diagnosis is based on finding *Schistosoma* eggs in the faeces, urine or, most reliably, in a rectal or bladder biopsy. Serology may be helpful in difficult cases or asymptomatic infection.

Treatment: A single dose of praziquantel.

BIBLIOGRAPHY AND FURTHER READING

Bacteria

Cohen, J.I., Bartlett, J.A. & Corey, G.R. (1987). Extra-intestinal manifestations of *Salmonella* infections. *Medicine* **66**:349–88.

Cohen, M.B. & Gianella, R.A. (1992). Hemorrhagic colitis associated with *Escherichia coli* 0157:H7. *Adv. Intern. Med.* **37**:173–95.

Doyle, M.P. (1991). *Escherichia coli* 0157:H7 and its significance in foods. *Internat. J. Food. Microbiol.* **12**:289–302.

Feeney, G.F.X., Kerlin, P. & Sampson, J.A. (1987). Clinical aspects of infection with *Yersinia enterocolitica* in adults. *Aust. N.Z. J. Med.* **17**:216–9.

Giannella, R.A., Broitman, S.A. & Zamchek, N. (1971). Salmonella enteritis. I. Role of reduced gastric secretion in pathogenesis. *Am. J. Dig. Dis.* **16**:1000–6.

Glass, R.I., Claeson, M., Blake, P.A., Waldman, R.J. & Pierce, N.F. (1991). Cholera in Africa: lessons on transmission and control for Latin America. *Lancet* **338**:791–5.

Griffin, P.H., Ostroff, S.M., Tauxe, R.V. et al. (1988). Illness associated with *Escherichia coli* 0157:H7 infections. A broad clinical spectrum. *Ann. Intern. Med.* **109**:705–12.

Haboubi, N.Y. & Montgomery, R.D. (1992). Small bowel bacterial overgrowth in elderly people: clinical significance and response to treatment. *Age Ageing* **21**:1–4.

Pentland, B. & Pennington, C.R. (1986). Acute diarrhoea in the elderly. *Age Ageing* **9**:90–2.

Portnoy, D.A. & Smith, G.A. (1992). Devious devices of Salmonella. *Nature* **357**:536.

Rybolt, A.H., Bennett, R.G., Laughon, B.E., Thomas, D.R., Greenough, W.B. III & Bartlett, J.G. (1989). Protein-losing enteropathy associated with *Clostridium difficile* infection. *Lancet* **1**:1353–5.

Saebo, A. & Lassen, J. (1991). Acute and chronic gastrointestinal manifestations associated with *Yersinia enterocolitica* infection. A Norwegian follow-up study on 458 hospitalized patients. *Ann. Surg.* **215**:250–5.

Parasites

Aristizabal, H., Acevedo, J. & Botero, M. (1991). Fulminant amebic colitis. *World J. Surg.* **15**:216–21.

Farthing, M.J.G. (1988). Tropical gastroenterology. In *Recent Advances in Gastroenterology*, ed. R.E. Pounder, pp. 177–96. Edinburgh: Churchill Livingstone.

Grove, D.I. (1991). Diarrhoea due to parasites. In *Diarrhoea*, ed. M. Gracey, pp. 93–113. BocaRaton, Boston: CRC Press Inc.

Lindsay, D.S., Dubey, J.P. & Blagburn, B.L. (1997). Biology of *Isospora spp.* from humans, non-human primates and domestic animals. *Clin. Microbiol. Rev.* **10**:19–34.

Stenzel, D.J. & Boreham, P.F.L. (1996). *Blastocystis hominis* revisited. *Clin. Microbiol. Rev.* **9**:563–84.

Trier, J.S., Moxey, P.C., Schimmel, E.M. & Robles, E. (1974). Chronic intestinal coccidiosis in man: Intestinal morphology and response to treatment. *Gastroenterol* **66**:923–35.

Winsland, J.K.D., Nimmo, S., Butcher, P.D. & Farthing, M.J. (1989). Prevalence of Giardia in dogs and cats in the United Kingdom: survey of an Essex veterinary clinic. *Trans. R. Soc. Trop. Med. Hyg.* **83**:791–2

Wittner, M. & Tanowitz, H.B. (1992). Intestinal parasites in returned travelers. *Med. Clin. North Am.* **76**:1433–48.

Yoon, J.H., Ryu, J.G., Lee, J.K. et al. (1991). Atypical clinical manifestations of amebic colitis. *J. Korean Med. Sci.* **6**:260–6.

Viruses

Augustin, A.K., Simon, A.E., Shorrock, C. & McCausland, J. (1995). Outbreaks of gastroenteritis due to Norwalk-like virus in two long-term care facilities for the elderly. *Can. J. Infect. Control* **10**:111–3.

Blacklow, N.R. & Greenberg, H.B. (1991). Viral gastroenteritis. *N. Engl. J. Med.* **325**:252–64.

Chadwick, P.R. & McCann, R. (1994). Transmission of a small round structured virus by vomiting during a hospital outbreak of gastroenteritis. *J. Hosp. Infect.* **26**:251–9.

Cubitt, W.D., Pead, P.J. & Saeed, A.A. (1981). A new type of Calicivirus associated with an outbreak of gastroenteritis in a residential home for the elderly. *J. Clin. Pathol.* **34**:924–6.

Dinulos, M.B. & Matson, D.O. (1994). Recent developments with human Caliciviruses. *Pediatr. Infect. Dis. J.* **13**:998–1003.

Escudero-Fabre, A., Cummings, O., Kirklin, J.K., Bourge, R.C. & Aldrete, J.S. (1992). Cytomegalovirus colitis presenting as hematochezia and requiring resection. *Arch. Surg.***127**:102–4.

Friedman, S.L. (1994). Diarrhoea. In *The AIDS Knowledge Base*, ed. P.T. Cohen, M.A. Sande & P.A. Volberding, pp. 5.19.1–5.19.19. Boston: Little Brown.

Guerrant, R.L. & Bobak, D.A. (1995) Nausea, vomiting and non-inflammatory diarrhoea. In *Principles and Practice of Infectious Diseases*, 4th edn, ed. G.L. Mandell, J.E. Bennett & R. Dolin, pp. 965–77. New York: Churchill Livingstone.

Lewis, D.C., Lightfoot, N.F., Cubitt, W.D. & Wilson, S.A. (1989). Outbreaks of Astrovirus type1 and Rotavirus gastroenteritis in a geriatric in-patient population. *J. Hosp. Infect.* **14**:9–14.

Marrie, T.J., Lee, S.H.S., Faulkner, R.S., Ethier, J & Young, C.H. (1982). Rotavirus infection in a geriatric population. *Arch. Intern. Med.* **142**:313–6.

Mitchell, E., O'Mahoney, M., McKeith, I., Sprott, M.S., Codd, A.A. & Wright, A.G. (1989). An outbreak of viral gastroenteritis in a psychiatric hospital. *J. Hosp. Infect.* **14**:1–8.

9   **Specific infectious conditions**

Ranjit N. Ratnaike

Bacterial overgrowth in the small intestine (blind loop syndrome, stagnant loop syndrome)

A form of diarrhoea peculiar to the elderly is associated with significant small bowel bacterial overgrowth. There is no evidence of systemic disease involving the small intestine nor anatomical abnormalities commonly associated with this entity (duodenal diverticula, small intestinal diverticulosis, surgical anastomoses, fistulas, strictures, mechanical obstructions). Bacterial overgrowth is reported to be a common cause of malabsorption in patients over the age of 80 years in whom there was no radiological or histological abnormality of the small intestine.

In the elderly, decreased nonimmunological and immunological defences of the gastrointestinal tract, discussed previously (see Chapters 1 and 2) predispose to bacterial overgrowth. The causes of hypomotility are systemic diseases and local conditions which involve the small intestine. The systemic conditions are hypothyroidism, diabetic autonomic neuropathy, amyloidosis, scleroderma and myotonia dystrophica. The local conditions include intestinal pseudo-obstruction, lymphoma and radiation enteritis.

Hypomotility due to hypothyroidism is perhaps not sufficiently recognized as a potential cause of bacterial overgrowth of the small intestine in the elderly. In a recent study on a group of elderly hypothyroid patients on thyroxine, the median orocaecal transit time increased from 75 to 135 minutes when thyroxine was withdrawn.

Another cause of bacterial overgrowth is intestinal pseudo-obstruction. This condition is often idiopathic although secondary causes are well documented (see Chapter 15).

Bacterial overgrowth of the small intestine results in diarrhoea due to deconjugation of the primary bile salts (the glycine and taurine conjugates of cholic and chenodeoxycholic acid) by bacterial enzymes. This leads to the formation of secondary bile acids, predominantly deoxycholic acid, which promote net fluid and electrolyte secretion in the colon through: (1) decreased water absorption; (2)

114

increased secretion of fluids and electrolytes; and (3) increased motor activity, which contribute to diarrhoea. Diarrhoea may also result from impaired fat absorption in the small intestine due to decreased micelle formation. Undigested dietary components may act as organic solutes to cause osmotic diarrhoea.

The common consequences of bacterial overgrowth are malabsorption of nutrients, minerals and vitamins resulting in steatorrhoea and megaloblastic anaemia due to vitamin B_{12} deficiency.

The definitive diagnosis is by a bacterial count greater than 10^6 in a sterile aspirate of duodenal or jejunal fluid. A more convenient diagnostic test is the ^{14}C-xylose breath test (see Chapter 5).

With regard to treatment, the underlying condition which predisposes to bacterial overgrowth should be treated if practicable. In patients with no demonstrable cause, as in many elderly patients, a course of antibiotics is recommended, given in cycles to prevent further bacterial overgrowth and antibiotic resistance. Tetracycline and erythromycin are commonly used. Antibiotic therapy ultimately resolves the problems of malabsorption and undernutrition.

Tropical sprue

Tropical sprue is a primary malabsorption syndrome in residents or visitors to certain areas of the tropics. An epidemic of tropical sprue has been reported in South India. Both the epidemiological features and the response to tetracycline therapy point to an infective aetiology in this condition.

An important distinction from coeliac disease is that in tropical sprue the entire small intestine is involved and both folate and vitamin B_{12} absorption is impaired. In coeliac disease ileal damage is rare and, hence, decreased vitamin B_{12} absorption is unusual.

The symptoms consist of malaise and easy fatiguability, weight loss, diarrhoea and abdominal discomfort. Bowel movements are typical of steatorrhoea and are of large volume, offensive and difficult to flush away. The elderly may present initially with severe anaemia and cardiac failure due to combined folate and B_{12} deficiency.

Histological findings of the small intestine show villous atrophy and an inflammatory infiltrate of the lamina propria.

Biochemical investigations reflect malabsorption. The d-xylose excretion test is abnormal; the three-day faecal fat is elevated. In some patients with tropical sprue folate concentrations are not reduced; steatorrhoea is not universal. The possibility that differences such as these have a geographical basis has been mooted.

The main purpose of radiological investigation of the small intestine in tropical sprue, as in other malabsorptive states, is to rule out an anatomical abnormality. There are no radiological features diagnostic of tropical sprue.

Thus the radiological features listed below reflect severe malabsorption of small mucosal bowel origin irrespective of the aetiology. The small intestine is dilated. The abnormal appearances of barium in the small intestine include:

- flocculation of barium (the barium is seen as large clumps obscuring the intestine)
- fragmentation of barium (this gives a mottled appearance)
- puddling of barium (residual barium in the mucosal folds after the passage of the barium)
- segmentation (lengths of bowel with no barium are seen between areas with barium)
- the moulage sign (obliteration of mucosal folds).

In making the diagnosis of tropical sprue it is important to exclude parasitic causes of malabsorption, especially *giardiasis* (see Chapter 8).

Therapy consists of correcting the nutritional consequences of malabsorption. Specific treatment for tropical sprue is a combination of folic acid and tetracycline, usually for several months until there is evidence of histological improvement of small intestine morphology.

Whipple's disease

Whipple's disease is a rare, multisystem illness thought to occur usually in middle aged white males. However, a recent review by Durand et al. (1997) of 52 patients reported an age range at the time of diagnosis of 20–80 years (mean 55 years). The mean age at diagnosis was 50 years for male patients and 58 years for female patients. In Whipple's disease the dominant symptoms related to the gastrointestinal tract, and malabsorption and weight loss are prominent features.

Recently, the gram-positive, periodic acid-Schiff (PAS)-positive bacillus associated with the disease has been identified using the polymerase chain reaction (PCR). The causative organism has been named *Tropheryma whipplei*.

Diarrhoea, due to gastrointestinal tract involvement, and arthritis are dominant features. Arthritis may precede intestinal symptoms by months or years. The knees and ankles are commonly affected. Involvement of the central nervous system and the heart, due to infiltration by macrophages, also occurs. Leucocytosis and occasional eosinophilia are present. The diagnosis is made on the uniquely diagnostic small bowel biopsy which shows the lamina propria laden with PAS-positive foamy macrophages and bacteria. Small intestinal villous abnormalities are variable.

The procedure for diagnosis has been a small bowel biopsy with evidence of PAS-positive macrophages infiltrating the lamina propria and the presence of bacilliform organisms best demonstrable on electron microscopy. The PCR has been shown to be the diagnostic tool of choice. The test is highly sensitive and specific and is now invaluable not only in diagnosis but also to monitor the patient's response to treatment. The role of PCR as a tool for monitoring is especially important as relapse occurs in about a third of patients treated with antibiotics.

Treatment with penicillin and streptomycin for two weeks and trimethoprim-sulfamethoxazole for 12 months is recommended to produce a complete remission.

Despite the rarity of the condition, Whipple's disease is a diagnosis worth pursuing in patients in whom the diagnosis of diarrhoea is elusive. The failure to diagnose and treat Whipple's disease results in death.

Traveller's diarrhoea

Travel abroad is increasing in popularity especially with the fit, affluent elderly. The risk of acquiring traveller's diarrhoea depends on the destination of travel. Geographical areas are designated according to the potential risk they pose to visitors:

- high risk – Africa; Latin America; Asia
- moderate risk – Southern Europe; Middle East; some Caribbean islands; China
- low risk – Northern Europe; North America; Australia and New Zealand; Japan; some Caribbean Islands.

On the information available, the chance of a traveller from a developed country acquiring diarrhoea during travel to a high risk area is 20 to 50 per cent, although the standard of hygiene may differ markedly in a particular geographical region or a single country.

Traveller's diarrhoea is less likely to occur in the elderly traveller who is likely to indulge in a less adventurous dietary style and opt for better accommodation than a younger tourist who may eat in cheaper restaurants and live in inexpensive accommodation where lavatories are shared and hygiene is not optimal.

Traveller's diarrhoea can be a nuisance at the best of times; or a memorable misadventure. Euphemisms for traveller's diarrhoea abound: Aztec two step, Delhi belly, Ho Chi Minh's, Hong Kong dog, Montezuma's revenge, Rangoon runs, seeping slickness, tourist trots, and Turkey trots.

The cause of diarrhoea is not always an infection. Noninfective causes include:

- overindulgence of free airline food and drink
- fear of flying and thoughts of the return flight
- overindulgence of local fruit
- the stress of living abroad; delays; frustrations; not being in control; problems with travel companions
- spicy food, e.g. hot curries.

The aetiology of diarrhoea is known in only 80 per cent of patients despite intense study. The evidence points to bacteria, protozoa and helminths as the major cause of traveller's diarrhoea (see Chapter 9). The common pathogens causing traveller's diarrhoea include bacteria, parasites and viruses (see Chapter 9).

The common causative bacteria are:

- enterotoxigenic *E. coli* (ETEC)
- enteroadherent *E. coli* (EAEC)
- enteroinvasive *E. coli* (EIEC)
- Salmonella sp.
- Shigella sp.
- *Campylobacter jejuni*
- *Aeromonas hydrophila.*

The parasites consist of *Giardia lamblia, Entamoeba histolytica, Cryptosporidium,* and *Strongyloides stercoralis.* Rotavirus is the most frequent viral agent.

Enterotoxigenic *E. coli* (ETEC) is the most common aetiological agent. The symptoms of diarrhoea vary with the pathogen. Diarrhoea of a secretory nature with watery motions and no evidence of blood in the stools occurs with enterotoxigenic *E. coli* (ETEC), enteroadherent *E. coli* (EAEC), *Cryptosporidium* and Rotavirus. Dysentery is a feature of infectious *Shigella* sp., especially *S. dysenteriae* type 1 and enteroinvasive *E. coli* (EIEC). *Aeromonas hydrophila* and the protozoan parasite *Cryptosporidium* are identified increasingly as aetiological agents in traveller's diarrhoea. As more sophisticated laboratory techniques for the identification of enteric pathogens are developed, 'newer' pathogens could be identified.

The aetiology of traveller's diarrhoea varies with the geographical area. *Giardia* and *Cryptosporidium* are frequent causes of diarrhoea in tourists who visit St. Petersburg (Leningrad), Russia. *Salmonella* sp. are commonly acquired during travel in the Indian subcontinent and southern Asia. In Thailand and Bangladesh *Campylobacter jejuni* is a more common cause of traveller's diarrhoea than in Mexico where *E. coli* (ETEC) is frequently isolated.

Travellers to areas of inadequate hygiene and sanitation should take sensible steps to prevent infection, summed up by the advice: 'if you can't peel it, shell it, boil it or cook it, don't eat it.' Depending on where one travels, finding food to satisfy these criteria may not be easy. Consuming boiled or cooked food for breakfast, lunch and dinner is not to everyone's taste and in most developing countries 'safe' 'western food' is not easy to obtain; if available it is expensive. It is safe to drink bottled carbonated beverages, hot tea, coffee, water boiled or treated with chlorine or iodine, and alcohol such as local beer.

Dietary items to especially avoid are dairy products, raw sea food, unpeeled raw fruit, and fruit and vegetable salads. Foods that may have been cooked and left unrefrigerated should not be eaten. Food from street vendors is associated with a high degree of enteric infections. Western visitors to developing countries often forget that refrigeration is expensive, power supplies capricious and the quantity of water available to practice optimal hygiene is limited. There is no guarantee that tap water is safe water. The most meticulous travellers who drink only bottled water may unwittingly 'slip up' adding ice to bottled water or bottled soft drinks; eat a salad; and have a milk-based local confectionary, ice cream or fruit salad for dessert. The traveller should not be lulled into being less wary of enteric infection by the grand appearance of a hotel building and its liveried staff or if the establishment belongs to a chain they are familiar with and for which they have a high regard.

The question of prophylaxis is important. The elderly, especially those who are more likely to acquire diarrhoea should be advised to consider the risks of diarrhoea before travel. Those with cardiovascular, renal or liver disease on diurectics are especially susceptible to dehydration and electrolyte depletion – more so if the weather is hot. Nausea and vomiting and malabsorption of prescribed medicine is another hazard.

In the elderly, one approach is to provide prophylaxis to patients with concurrent illnesses that would significantly worsen due to diarrhoea, or have an adverse effect on the medication they take due to dehydration and haemoconcentration, or malabsorption of the medication. The elderly, in whom immunological and nonimmunological defences may be depressed due to illness or drug therapy, would also benefit from prophylaxis.

Advice should be given on how to minimize the risk of diarrhoea and what steps should be taken if diarrhoea occurs. The dangers of dehydration, and its prevention, should be thoroughly discussed. A plan of action should be decided on before departure. While abroad the importance of seeking early medical attention, particularly for dysentery or for more than four bowel actions a day, or for vomiting, must be discussed. Should the patient's physician be contacted? If this is agreed on, under what circumstances should this be done? It may be possible to furnish the traveller with the name(s) of a medical practitioner in the places to be visited. If the elderly traveller carries drugs for the treatment of diarrhoea on the advice of the physician, the indication for their use, dosage and side effects should be clearly understood. Oral rehydration salts (ORS) packets can be carried and reconstituted when required.

A popular prophylactic agent for traveller's diarrhoea is bismuth subsalicylate. Extensive studies have demonstrated its efficacy as a prophylactic agent against traveller's diarrhoea. One view regarding prophylactic antibiotics, based on cost-effectiveness studies, is that their use is justified: in addition to benefits to health, travel is not disrupted and additional expense is not incurred nor time wasted. These advantages have to be weighed against the possibility of adverse drug reactions and the emergence of resistant organisms. Suitable antimicrobials for prophylaxis are trimethoprim-sulfamethoxazole, norfloxacin and ciprofloxacin.

Deoxycycline is no longer recommended due to resistant enterotoxigenic *E. coli* (ETEC), *Salmonella* sp. and *Shigella* sp.

The traveller should also be advised against the purchase of over-the-counter medication for diarrhoea and to be extremely cautious of therapy prescribed locally. The sale of drugs which are ineffective and expensive is widespread in the developing world. Compounds prescribed for diarrhoea such as iodochlorhydroxyquin (Enterovioform, Elioquinol) and other halogenated hydroxyquinolone derivatives have dubious therapeutic value but are established causes of myelo-optic neuropathy.

Treatment

If diarrhoea occurs the patient should be advised to increase fluid intake. In addition to carbonated soft drinks, commercially available oral rehydration solutions should be used.

Antimotility drugs such as loperamide or diphenoxylate, provide effective relief of symptoms. Contraindications are fever, and blood and mucus in the stools, or if the diarrhoea continues for longer than 48 hours.

Antibiotics are indicated in patients with dysentery or if the diarrhoea persists for longer than 48 hours. Whether an antibiotic should be taken earlier should be discussed with the physician before travel. The antibiotics which may be used are: trimethoprim-sulfamethoxazole, norfloxacin and ciprofloxacin.

In patients with chronic diarrhoea after travel abroad, the possibility of a parasitic infection, especially *Giardia lamblia* (since the incubation period is 14 to 21 days), should be vigorously pursued.

Diarrhoea associated with AIDS

Patients with AIDS are especially vulnerable to enteric infections due to the depletion of CD4+ cells which are involved in the primary immune response of the small intestine.

The prevalence of diarrhoea in patients with AIDS varies from 30 to 80 per cent, and a pathogen is identified in up to 80 per cent of patients. Often, patients are infected with multiple pathogens. The most common organisms identified in faeces are *Cryptosporidium*, *Mycobacterium avium intracellulare*, *Clostridium difficile* and *Isospora belli*. The frequent enteric pathogens associated with diarrhoea in patients with AIDS are Cytomegalovirus and Herpes simplex virus; fungi such as *Candida* sp.; and bacteria such as *Mycobacterium avium intracellulare (MAI)*, *Salmonella* sp., *Shigella* sp., *Campylobacter jejuni*, *Clostridium difficile*, and *Aeromonas hydrophila*. Parasitic infections are commonly due to *Giardia lamblia*,

Entamoeba histolytica, Cryptosporidium, Microsporidium, Isospora belli, Sarcocystis hominis and *Strongyloides stercoralis*.

Diarrhoea associated with AIDS is not invariably due to an enteric infection since pathogens are isolated from faeces in the absence of diarrhoea. Other aetiological factors such as a malignancy or the side-effect of drug therapy should be considered. Drugs such as opiates, loperamide and diphenoxylate may be of symptomatic value.

AIDS enteropathy

In recent times attention has focused on AIDS enteropathy characterized by chronic diarrhoea of unknown aetiology. The role, if any, of HIV-1 infection as the primary or contributory cause of the enteropathy is as yet unclear. The clinical picture is one of weight loss, malabsorption and profuse diarrhoea refractory to symptomatic therapy with antimotility drugs. Small intestinal villous changes are a frequent and prominent feature.

A major recent advance in the control of diarrhoea is the use of octreotide, a synthetic, long-acting octapeptide analogue of somatostatin. The rationale for using the drug is based on the physiological actions of somatostatin which stimulates the small intestinal epithelial cells to absorb Na, Cl and water and to decrease Cl secretion. The overall result is net fluid absorption.

BIBLIOGRAPHY AND FURTHER READING

Bacterial overgrowth in the small intestine

Haboubi, N.Y. & Montgomery, R.D. (1992). Small bowel bacterial overgrowth in elderly people: clinical significance and response to treatment. *Age Ageing* 21:13–9.

Holt, P. (1992). Clinical significance of bacterial overgrowth in elderly people. *Age Ageing* 21:1–4.

Lipski, P.S., Kelly, P.J. & James, O.F. (1992). Bacterial contamination of the small bowel in elderly people: is it necessarily pathological? *Age Ageing* 21:5–12.

McEvoy, A., Dutton, J. & James, O.F. (1983). Bacterial contamination of the small intestine is an important cause of occult malabsorption in the elderly. *Br. Med. J. Clin. Res. Ed.* 287:789–93.

Montgomery, R.O., Haboubi, N.Y., Mike, N.H., Chesner, I.M. & Asquith, P. (1986). Causes of malabsorption in the elderly. *Age Ageing* 15:235–40.

Rahman, Q., Haboubi, N.Y., Hudson, P.R., Lee, G.S. & Shah, I.U. (1991) The effect of thyroxine on small intestinal motility in the elderly. *Clin. Endocrinol.* 35:443–6.

Tropical sprue

Klipstein, F.A. (1981). Tropical sprue in travelers and expatriates living abroad. *Gastroenterology* 80:590–600.

Mathan, V.I. & Baker, S.J. (1970). An epidemic of tropical sprue in southern India. I. Clinical features. *Ann. Trop. Med. Parasitol.* **64**:439–51.

Tomkins, A. (1986). Tropical sprue and tropical enteropathy. In *Infections of the Gastrointestinal Tract*, ed. P.D. Manuel, J.A. Walker-Smith & A. Tomkins, pp. 212–34. Edinburgh: Churchill Livingstone.

Whipple's disease

Donaldson, R.M. Jr. (1992). Whipple's disease – a rare malady with uncommon potential. *N. Engl. J. Med.* **327**:346–8.

Durand, D.V., Lecomte, C., Cathebras, P., Rousset, H., Godeau, P., SNFMI Research Group on Whipple Disease (1997). Whipple disease. Clinical review of 52 Cases. *Medicine* **76**:170–84.

Fleming, J.L., Wiesner, R.H. & Shorter, R.G. (1988). Whipple's disease: clinical, biochemical and histopathologic features and assessment of treatment in 29 patients. *Mayo. Clin. Proc.* **63**:539–51.

Ramzan, N.N., Loftus, E. Jr, Burgart, L.J. et al. (1997). Diagnosis and monitoring of Whipple disease by polymerase chain reaction. *Ann. Intern. Med.* **126**:520–7.

Relman, D.A., Schmidt, T.M., MacDermott, R.P. & Falkow, S. (1992). Identification of the uncultured bacillus of Whipple's disease. *N. Engl. J. Med.* **327**:293–301.

Whipple, G.H. (1907). A hitherto undescribed disease characterised anatomically by deposits of fat and fatty acids in the intestinal and mesenteric lymphatic tissues. *Bull Johns Hopkins Hosp.* **18**:382–91.

Traveller's diarrhoea

Gorbach, S.L. (1992). Traveler's diarrhoea. In *Infectious Diseases,* ed. S.L. Gorbach, J.G. Bartlett & N.R. Blacklow, pp. 622–8. Philadelphia: Saunders.

Looke, D.F. (1990). Traveller's diarrhoea. *Aust. Fam. Physician* **19**:194–203.

Okhuysen, P.C. & Ericsson, C.D. (1992). Traveler's diarrhoea. Prevention and treatment. *Med. Clin. North Am.* **76**:1357–73.

Diarrhoea associated with AIDS

Bartlett, J.G., Belitsos, P.C. & Sears, C.L. (1992). AIDS enteropathy. *Clin. Infect. Dis.* **15**:726–35.

Cello, J.P., Grendell, J.H., Basuk, P. et al. (1991). Effect of octreotide on refractory AIDS-associated diarrhoea. *Ann. Intern. Med.* **115**:705–10.

Fanning, M., Monte, M., Sutherland, L.R., Broadhead, M., Murphy, G.F. & Harris, A.G. (1991). Pilot study of Sandostatin (Octreotide) therapy of refractory HIV-associated diarrhoea. *Dig. Dis. Sci.* **36**:476–80.

Smith, P.D., Quinn, T.C., Strober, W., Janoff, E.N. & Masur, H. (1992) NIH Conference. Gastrointestinal infections in AIDS. *Ann. Intern. Med.* **116**:63–77.

Tanowitz, H.B., Simon, D. & Wittner, M. (1992) Medical management of AIDS patients. Gastrointestinal manifestations. *Med. Clin. North Am.* **76**:45–62.

10 An overview of management of infectious diarrhoea

Ranjit N. Ratnaike

Most enteric infections cause mild diarrhoea and no therapy is necessary in healthy individuals. Diarrhoea should be regarded with caution in the elderly who are more susceptible to the complications of even a single episode of acute diarrhoea. The elderly with an illness coexistent at the time of diarrhoea are at even greater risk.

In the management of diarrhoea a sensible balance has to be struck between unnecessary treatment and neglect on the part of both the physician and patient. With regard to the healthy elderly, medical advice should be sought if a circumstance listed below occurs:

- bloody diarrhoea
- abdominal pain and tenderness, rectal pain, tenesmus
- persistent vomiting and inability to retain fluids for a six-hour period
- fever
- evidence of dehydration
- more than five to six bowel actions in 24 hours
- patients with current medical problems
- patients on drug therapy.

The frail, debilitated elderly and patients on medication should be advised to contact their physician at the onset of diarrhoea.

The patient (and/or care-giver) should be instructed about the need for increased fluid intake and a plan agreed on further intervention. The extent of involvement of the physician and treatment would depend on the nature and course of the diarrhoeal illness and the state of the patient's existing clinical status. Guidelines for advice during an episode of diarrhoea at home are:

- decrease physical activity
- stay indoors on a hot day
- drink plenty of fluids (up to three litres per day, unless there is a contraindication)
- avoid milk and alcohol
- do not stop eating solids; eat what can be tolerated
- avoid milk products; high roughage food; spicy food; raw food
- take a drug such as loperamide if recommended by your physician

- avoid home remedies unless they are first discussed with your doctor
- wash hands frequently, especially after going to the toilet, before eating and before handling oral medication.

Care should be taken to ensure that the patient or care-giver understands the instructions given. Written instructions which are easy to read and understand are useful in addition to those given verbally.

The prevention of dehydration and electrolyte loss should be the primary management objective. The susceptibility to these complications and their consequences increases with age. These problems are compounded by existing illnesses, and diuretic therapy for cardiac failure or decompensated liver or renal disease.

In secretory diarrhoea major fluid loss of many litres per day may occur. Outputs of 15 l/day have been reported in patients with diarrhoea due to *V. cholerae*. In addition to fluid, loss of Na and K and, to a lesser extent, HCO_3 occurs. A less common complication is hyperchloraemic acidosis.

Assessment of dehydration

In assessing dehydration in the elderly the conventional criteria listed below are unreliable in the elderly patient. Gross et al. (1992) conducted a prospective, correlational study with 55 subjects aged 60 or older and concluded that these symptoms or signs were *not* strong correlates of dehydration in the elderly. This is due to the fact that these variables, in the elderly, reflect *normal age-related changes.* In addition, the physiological response to dehydration varies markedly between the elderly and younger patients. For example, postural hypotension is a common sign in the elderly patient, independent of the state of hydration, due to autonomic dysfunction and drug therapy.

Conventional criteria
- reduction of skin turgor
- increased thirst
- decreased peripheral perfusion
- postural hypotension
- low jugular venous pressure
- patient sensations of thirst and dryness
- tachycardia and elevated temperature.

Recommended criteria
Seven signs and symptoms are highlighted that strongly correlate with dehydration in the elderly, but are independent of significant, age-related change. They are:
- dry tongue
- longitudinal tongue furrows

- dry mucous membranes of nose and mouth
- eyes that appeared recessed in their sockets
- upper body muscle weakness
- speech difficulty
- confusion.

Rehydration

Oral rehydration alone is an effective means of fluid and electrolyte replacement in nearly all cases of dehydration. Most patients are able to maintain their hydration by increasing their intake of fluids such as water, mineral water, fruit juice and soft drinks. There is a possibility that large quantities of some drinks may impose a high osmotic load. Thus, in treating dehydration it is advisable to avoid fluids with a high osmolality such as Coca Cola (680 mOsm/kg), apple juice (870 mOsm/kg), orange juice (935 mOsm/kg) and grape juice (1170 mOsm/kg).

In clinical practice the problem with elderly patients is motivating them to take sufficient fluids. The decreased fluid intake is due to a variety of causes and includes:

- a decreased perception of thirst
- inability to ask for fluids due to dementia or altered consciousness
- physical inability to obtain fluids
- inability to drink because of dysphagia
- reluctance to drink because of fear of nocturia or incontinence.

Drinks containing caffeine have a diuretic action and should be avoided. Elderly patients may have to be actively encouraged to increase their fluid intake. The rationale for the effectiveness of oral rehydration solutions is that, despite severe diarrhoea, the mechanisms of Na and water absorption are not impaired. The presence of glucose in the solution allows the entry of Na into the intestinal epithelial cell. This process, termed cotransport, in a simplistic sense results in Na being 'piggy backed' on a glucose molecule.

Intravenous therapy is often used more as a convenience than a therapeutic necessity. In a proportion of elderly patients dehydration may be associated with confusion and oral intake may be difficult to maintain, thus requiring intravenous fluids. Intravenous therapy should be given to patients in shock, with hypovolaemia and those with persistent vomiting or problems of deglutition.

Nutrition

Undernutrition is a common problem in the elderly. In episodes of both acute and, especially, chronic diarrhoea the nutritional status of the patient should be carefully assessed. Diarrhoea can lead to decreased food intake, impaired nutrient absorption and increased protein loss. Protein loss during diarrhoea is a major problem in the elderly and may continue during convalescence. Malnutrition can easily result, more so when the diarrhoea occurs during another serious, debilitating illness or when the patient's nutritional status before the diarrhoea is inadequate.

Chapter 18 deals extensively with the important relationship between diarrhoea and nutrition.

Diarrhoea is not an indication for fasting. The notion that 'rest is best for the gut' is without foundation. The view that what goes in through the mouth comes out as a diarrhoeal motion, although incorrect, is widely held. The duration of diarrhoeal episodes is reduced if nutrients and fluids and electrolytes are available for epithelial cell regeneration when mucosal damage has occurred. In the elderly, in whom undernutrition or malnutrition is often an existing problem, fasting during an episode of diarrhoea can seriously worsen the state of nutrition. Patients should be encouraged to eat food that can be tolerated. Foods to avoid are those with a high fat content or with a high roughage content, spicy food and raw food.

Antibiotics

The rationale for the cautious use of antibiotics in diarrhoea is well founded. Many enteric pathogens cause a self-limiting acute episode of diarrhoea. Viruses which do not respond to antibiotics are a common cause of diarrhoea. Susceptibility of most bacterial pathogens to antibiotics is highly specific for individual organisms. The clinical response to antibiotics may not parallel in vitro activity against the organism and resistant strains may emerge during treatment. Even worse, antibiotic treatment may induce antibiotic-associated diarrhoea separate from pseudomembraneous colitis, as well as other adverse effects.

Newer antibiotics such as ciprofloxacin and norfloxacin allay some of these concerns and have a broad spectrum of activity against the most common and important pathogens that cause dysentery.

The decision whether or not to use antibiotics depends on the severity of the diarrhoea and the current clinical circumstances of the patient, and should take into account the potential side-effects. Antibiotics are indicated in dysentery, especially if systemic symptoms such as fever, chills, headache and myalgia are present. Treatment with antibiotics should be directed to the specific pathogen identified on stool culture. In the period before the results of stool culture are available, if treatment is considered necessary the choice of antibiotic should be based on the clinical picture and knowledge of the pathogens which commonly cause diarrhoea in the local setting: in these circumstances, trimethoprim-sulfamethoxazole, norfloxacin or, if systemic symptoms are prominent, ciprofloxacin. The possibility of a parasitic cause of dysentery, such as *Entamoeba histolytica,* would have to be ruled out before antibiotic treatment is initiated.

Antimotility drugs

Antimotility drugs such as opiates, loperamide and diphenoxylate delay the passage of the intestinal contents. This allows more time for fluid and electrolyte absorption.

Loperamide is the drug of choice and is now available as an over-the-counter agent in 110 countries. A number of major studies which compared the efficacy and side-effects of loperamide concluded that it was superior to placebo, diphenoxylate and bismuth subsalicylate. The criteria for efficacy included the dose, stool frequency and consistency. The side-effects of loperamide are mild and temporary. In one report, a patient with ulcerative colitis treated with loperamide developed toxic megacolon. The use of the drug is not recommended in inflammatory bowel disease, infective diarrhoea with features of dysentery, and if fever or systemic toxic symptoms are present. Loperamide is a safe, effective drug in acute nonspecific diarrhoea. The suggested dose regime is 8 mg in 24 hours.

Adsorbents

Neither kaolin nor related compounds are effective in the treatment of diarrhoea. Kaolin absorbs water and increases the consistency of the stool but does not decrease the number of motions per day. It is suggested that bacteria and bacterial toxin may also be absorbed.

Bismuth subsalicylate (Pepto-Bismol), originally available as a liquid and now in tablet form, is a prophylactic agent in traveller's diarrhoea. The drug is a trivalent bismuth compound. On dissociation the bismuth forms salts which adversely affect bacterial metabolism, and the salicylate is absorbed. The recommended duration of use is three weeks. The contraindications are similar to those for aspirin. Since blood salicylate levels may be high, the concurrent ingestion of aspirin is not advised.

Antisecretory agents

Octreotide, an analogue of somatostatin, has been of value in the treatment of secretory diarrhoea due to *Cryptosporidium* and *Microsporidium* in patients with AIDS enteropathy (see Chapter 9). This compound has the potential to be widely used in patients with secretory diarrhoea.

The prevention of diarrhoea

Preventive aspects are often not sufficiently explained and emphasized to the elderly and their care-givers. These aspects range from personal, domestic and institutional hygiene, to food preparation and storage. In institutional settings both staff and patients should participate in learning that energetic preventive measures are needed to prevent the spread of infection.

The elderly patients who reside in a nursing home, rest home or geriatric ward are at a greater risk of acquiring diarrhoea, as a result of a point-source food-borne outbreak or due to person-to-person spread. The patients most at risk are those who are immunocompromised, those whose personal hygiene is suboptimal due to a physical or mental infirmity, and patients who are highly dependent on staff. Prompt action is required to prevent the spread of infection.

It is important to inform public health authorities immediately to document the outbreak, determine the source and the mode of transmission, identify the aetiological agent, if possible, and help with control measures.

The control of the spread of diarrhoea in a single ward is often difficult due to over-crowding, faecal incontinence, inadequate staff, and sharing common toilet facilities which are often inadequate. Measures to stop the spread of diarrhoea to other wards should be the major objective. It is suggested that all patients and staff from the 'infected ward' be restricted from entering other wards. A health education programme directed to patients and staff should be implemented and focused on:

- the thorough cleaning of toilets
- the meticulous disposal of faeces and soiled linen
- increased ward cleaning
- increased hand washing with soap, especially after visiting the toilet and before eating and handling medication
- optimal food handling practices.

Other precautions to take are to locate patients with diarrhoea near toilets. Staff with diarrhoea should be advised not to attend work, preferably until the pathogen which caused diarrhoea is no longer present in two consecutive stool samples.

With regard to food, patients at greatest risk of acquiring diarrhoea, for example those immunosuppressed, should avoid 'raw' milk and uncooked animal products. During cooking care should be taken to prevent the cross-contamination of cooked and fresh food, such as salads, from kitchen implements, utensils or surfaces used to prepare uncooked poultry, for example; this has the potential to harbour enteric pathogens.

Diarrhoea is now recognized as an important problem in the elderly by health professionals. Health education with regard to the prevention and management of diarrhoea and possible complications is an essential aspect of the care of the elderly. The elderly should be informed that diarrhoea may occur due to causes within the intestine, to systemic disease, and that it is a common side-effect of drug therapy.

It is important for patients and carers to appreciate that diarrhoea is often preventable and the complications of dehydration, electrolyte loss and undernutrition easily forestalled.

BIBLIOGRAPHY AND FURTHER READING

Bennett, R.G. & Greenough, W.B. III (1993). Approach to acute diarrhoea in the elderly. *Gastroenterol. Clin. North Am.* **22**:517–33.

Brown, J.W. (1979). Toxic megacolon associated with loperamide therapy. *J. Am. Med. Assoc.* **241**:501–2.

Dauterman, K.W., Bennett, R.G., Greenough, W.B. III et al. (1995). Plasma specific gravity for identifying hypovolaemia. *J. Diarrhoeal Dis. Res.* **13**:33–8.

Duepont, H.L., Flores-Sanchez, J.F., Ericsson, C.D. et al. (1990). Comparative efficacy of loperamide hydrochloride and bismuth subsalicylate in the management of acute diarrhoea. *Am. J. Med.* **88**:15S–19S.

Duepont, H.L. & Hornick, R.B. (1973). Adverse effect of lomotil therapy in shigellosis. *J. Am. Med. Assoc.* **226**:1525–8.

Ericsson, C.D. & Johnson, P.C. (1990). Safety and efficacy of loperamide. *Am. J. Med.* **88**:10S-14S.

Fanning, M., Monte, M., Sutherland, L.R., Broadhead, M., Murphy, G.F. & Harris, A.G. (1991). Pilot study of Sandostatin (Octreotide) therapy of refractory HIV-associated diarrhoea. *Dig. Dis. Sci.* **36**:476–80.

Fedorak, R.N. & Field, M. (1987). Antidiarrhoeal therapy, prospects for new agents. *Dig. Dis. Sci.* **32**:195–205.

Greenough, W.B. III & Khin-Maung, U. (1991). Oral rehydration therapy. In *Diarrhoeal Diseases*, ed. M. Field, pp. 485–499. New York: Elsevier.

Gross, C.R., Lindquist, R.D., Woolley, A.C., Granieri, R., Allard, K. & Webster, B. (1992). Clinical indicators of dehydration severity in elderly patients. *J. Emerg. Med.* **10**:267–74.

Neu, H.C. (1991). Antibiotics in the therapy of diarrhoea. In *Diarrhoeal Diseases*, ed. M. Field, pp. 441–54. New York: Elsevier.

Powell, D.W. (1991) Approach to the patient with diarrhoea. In *Textbook of Gastroenterology*, vol 1, ed. T. Yamada, pp. 732–78. Philadelphia: Lippincott.

Part III

Noninfectious clinical entities

Coeliac disease

Adrian G. Cummins

Introduction

It is not uncommon for coeliac disease to be diagnosed in elderly persons. Coeliac disease (synonyms: coeliac sprue, gluten-sensitive enteropathy) is a hypersensitivity reaction of the small intestine to the protein components of wheat, barley and rye cereals, which are all related in the same taxonomic tribe. This results in small intestinal damage in genetically predisposed individuals. It is a life-long disorder although the symptoms and age of presentation are variable. Patients with coeliac disease may present either after weaning or as adults. Teenagers with coeliac disease may notice that their symptoms remit and therefore they tend to default from their gluten-free diet, although it is known that their small bowel biopsies remain abnormal during this period. This temporary improvement during teenage years seems to explain the bimodal presentation that presumably depends on ileal compensation.

Coeliac disease, even when asymptomatic, may predispose to malabsorption of nutrients, metabolic bone disease and subsequent bone fractures, particularly in females, as well as to neoplasms such as intestinal lymphoma and adenocarcinoma, and head and oesophageal carcinomas. A high index of suspicion needs to be maintained such as requesting a duodenal biopsy during endoscopy examination for iron deficiency anaemia in the elderly. Often recurrent iron deficiency in this age group is wrongly attributed to colonic angiodysplasia, or to drugs such as nonsteroidal anti-inflammatory agents or warfarin.

Coeliac disease usually affects the proximal two-thirds of the small intestine where most of the nutrients are absorbed, except vitamin B_{12}, in the ileum. Intestinal damage leads to malabsorption of nutrients including carbohydrate, fats, proteins, vitamins and minerals.

The main toxic component is gluten, which is the major protein present in wheat. Other closely related cereals to wheat, such as rye and barley, contain similar toxic proteins. Proteins such as gluten are insoluble in water and soluble in 70 per cent ethanol. Gluten refers to the crude protein remaining after water extraction of milled wheat, while gliadin refers to the purified fraction of gluten that is soluble in 70 per cent ethanol.

Pathogenesis

A genetic predisposition is an absolute requirement for the expression of coeliac disease. Coeliac disease occurs in 70 per cent of identical twins and 10 per cent of first degree relatives. It is more common in Celtic (Irish, Scottish, Welsh), Scandinavian and Mediterranean ancestries. A major advance in recent years has been in defining this genetic predisposition in terms of human lymphocyte antigens (HLA), which are immune response genes that are best known in terms of organ transplantation.

In coeliac disease, the predisposing genes are DR3 or DR7, and DQ2 HLA antigens. About 80 to 90 per cent of coeliac patients of Northern European ancestry have the DR3 DQ2 genotype compared to 20–30 per cent of noncoeliac subjects. More than 95 per cent of coeliac subjects have the DQ2 haplotype. However, only about 0.1 per cent of subjects with these markers develop coeliac disease. The importance of these genes is that their corresponding peptide chains are located on the surface of antigen-presenting cells (macrophages and dendritic cells). Antigen binds in a specific shaped groove of the HLA peptide dimer and this complex then controls the activity of lymphocytes (Figure 11.1). It is the HLA–antigen complex that binds to the CD3 antigen receptor of the T lymphocyte.

It could be postulated that, in coeliac disease, gluten antigen either binds too well to cause uncontrolled overactivity of T lymphocytes, or it fails to bind to activate other suppressor T lymphocytes. Suppressor T lymphocytes normally suppress the overactivity of other delayed-type hypersensitivity T lymphocytes that presumably mediate the intestinal damage in coeliac disease. Some entities associated with coeliac disease are rheumatoid disease, type 1 diabetes mellitus, IgA nephropathy, isolated IgA deficiency, and autoimmune thyroid disease.

Clinical presentation

Symptoms

A high index of suspicion is needed to diagnose coeliac disease, as the classical symptoms of failure to thrive (babies) or weight loss (adults), chronic diarrhoea and malnutrition are uncommon. The classical symptoms of coeliac infants are a triad of failure to thrive, irritability and abdominal distension, but these are rarely seen these days. Adult subjects may have protean symptoms, such as diarrhoea or constipation, loss of weight, a bleeding disorder (especially in teenagers and young adults due to vitamin K deficiency), infertility, lethargy and shortness of breath, anaemia (iron or folate deficiency) and bone pain or fractures of metabolic bone disease (vitamin D deficiency). A progressive loss of weight in adults with a good appetite would suggest coeliac disease, although thyrotoxicosis needs to be

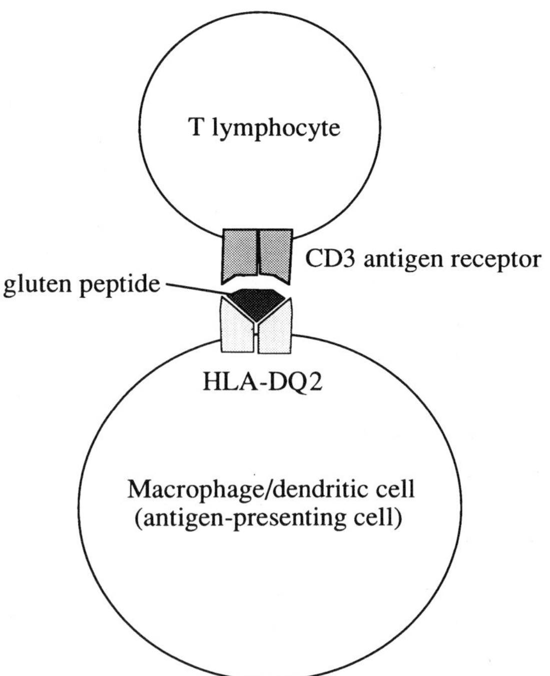

Figure 11.1. This diagram shows how antigen fits into the HLA–DQ2 molecule and this complex is presented to the CD3 antigen receptor of a T lymphocyte.

excluded. Coeliac patients older than 40 years may present with complicating neoplasms (see below).

Signs

Signs may be minimal. In a few cases, clubbing, ascites, ankle oedema and skin pigmentation may be present. Some patients may have aphthous mouth ulcers or associated dermatitis herpetiformis (itchy blistering vesicles on back and extensor surfaces). Specific features of mineral or vitamin deficiency may be present (glossitis, angular stomatitis, rash) but these are unusual. Older patients may have a glove and stocking sensory peripheral neuropathy, although this is common in many unaffected elderly patients.

Incidental presentation

Older patients may be found to have coeliac disease after initially being investigated for presumed gastrointestinal blood loss. Surgery of the gastrointestinal tract may render coeliac disease symptomatic. Some patients may present after being rejected as blood donors because of mild anaemia, or on referral to a physician because of a blood film showing features of splenic atrophy (Howell–Jolly bodies, acanthocytes, target cells and giant platelets). Coeliac disease may be diagnosed while investigating iron or folate deficiency anaemia, chronic gastric dilatation or other autonomic neuropathy, bleeding disorders, type 1 diabetes mellitus poorly responsive to insulin therapy, metabolic bone disease and fractures, and neoplasms.

Diagnosis

Intestinal biopsy is the primary investigation of coeliac disease and modern practice is to perform this as early as possible. The diagnosis of coeliac disease is made by a combination of abnormal serology with abnormal intestinal biopsy. It is important that this is done while the patient is still on a normal diet. It is now more convenient to take small bowel biopsies at endoscopy. When investigating iron deficiency anaemia in the elderly it is important to consider the possibility of coeliac disease. Elderly patients may undergo repeated endoscopy for iron deficiency of unknown origin without a duodenal biopsy being taken. A family history may give the clue to the diagnosis. Functional tests are seldom necessary (three-day faecal fats, xylose absorption) and only delay diagnosis.

The intestinal biopsy would show villous atrophy with surface effacement, crypt hyperplasia and increased intraepithelial lymphocytes. While these changes are not specific, they are useful when other causes of intestinal damage have been considered and excluded.

It is important to interpret an abnormal intestinal biopsy in combination with appropriate serology such as antigliadin IgA and IgG antibodies. Usually the antigliadin IgA titre will be higher than the IgG titre. Antigliadin IgA antibody is a suitable screening test for coeliac disease in first degree relatives or those with autoimmune diseases (rheumatoid disease, type 1 diabetes mellitus). Thus, siblings of coeliac subjects should be screened by an antigliadin IgA antibody test. The only limitation is coexisting IgA deficiency that may give a false negative result. IgA deficiency is associated with coeliac disease and indeed is believed to be an autoimmune disease. Measurement of antigliadin antibody is available in some major teaching hospitals, and as a commercial test kit. A high antigliadin IgA titre, however, does not diagnose coeliac disease, and should always be confirmed by an intestinal biopsy.

Three biopsies are recommended: the first to show intestinal damage; a second to show improvement on a gluten-free diet; and a third on gluten challenge to demonstrate that the previous improvement was specific and not coincidental. There is a more recent tendency to diagnose coeliac disease without gluten challenge. This is because it is easier to exclude other causes of villous atrophy such as giardiasis. However, there may be some adult patients where the diagnosis is in doubt and gluten challenge is necessary. Of course, it makes little sense to proceed with gluten challenge, if the patient is happy to tolerate a gluten-free diet indefinitely.

Treatment

As coeliac disease is an immunologically mediated disease, the treatment options are removal of the antigen by a gluten-free diet, or to suppress the overactivity of T lymphocytes by immunosuppressive agents (corticosteroids, cytotoxic agents, cyclosporin A). A gluten-free diet is a very difficult and bland diet, and it is arguable whether there is total gluten exclusion. This probably explains why the intestinal biopsy in adults rarely returns to normal. Gluten gives food elasticity and is present in may processed foods (including soups and gravies), and is used as a binding agent in some therapeutic medications. Rice and corn cause no toxicity and other toxic cereals may be substituted with soybean meal. The quality control of gluten-free cereals, such as are obtained from health food shops, may be variable. Suspect cereal batches can be tested by a gluten detection kit. A local coeliac society will be helpful in providing information on suitable foods and places of purchase. There is rarely the need to consider immunosuppression. Coincidental immunosuppression for other medical problems will, however, improve coeliac disease and may adversely increase absorption of medications and result in toxic levels.

Failure to improve on a gluten-free diet suggests either deliberate or accidental gluten ingestion, which may be determined by an antigliadin IgA antibody test.

Neoplasia of coeliac disease

Patients older than 40 years are at risk of presenting with, or developing, complicating neoplasia especially if they refuse to adhere to a gluten-free diet. However, individual patients with coeliac disease are only at about a two–fold increased risk of malignancy compared with normal subjects. A gluten-free diet for five years or greater (though imperfect) seems adequate in reducing the risk of neoplasia and controlling symptoms. The principal neoplasm is enteropathy-associated T cell lymphoma (EATCL), which was formerly termed malignant histiocytosis of the intestine. This is a specific malignancy of intraepithelial lymphocytes in coeliac disease. The relative risk is increased 70-fold in coeliac subjects who do not adhere to a gluten-free diet. Other neoplasia associated with coeliac disease are adenocarcinoma of the duodenum, oesophageal carcinoma, and head and neck carcinomas.

Other causes of malabsorption

Other conditions associated with malabsorption are:

- ulcerative jejunitis and intestinal lymphoma (EATCL) of coeliac disease

- cow's milk allergy and other food hypersensitivities (mainly infants and usually transient)
- giardiasis
- bacterial overgrowth (scleroderma or surgical blind loop)
- congenital immunodeficiencies
- HIV enteropathy
- graft-versus-host disease (after bone marrow transplantation)
- tropical sprue (rare)
- Whipple's disease (rare).

The early distinction between maldigestion of pancreatic origin and malabsorption of small bowel origin is important. Useful screening tests in pancreatic disease are ultrasound and CT scan. In some instances, ERCP (endoscopic retrograde cholangiopancreatogram) may be necessary. A small bowel cause of malabsorption is diagnosed by small intestinal biopsy (see Chapter 5).

BIBLIOGRAPHY AND FURTHER READING

Crabtree, J.E., Heatley, R.V., Juby, L.D., Howdle, P.D. & Losowsky, M.S. (1989). Serum interleukin-2 receptor in coeliac disease: response to treatment and gluten challenge. *Clin. Exp. Immunol.* 77:345–8.

Cummins, A.G., Penttila, I.A., LaBrooy, J.T., Robb, T.A. & Davidson, G.P. (1991). Recovery of the small intestine in coeliac disease on a gluten-free diet: changes in intestinal permeability, small bowel morphology and T-cell activity. *J. Gastroenterol Hepatol.* 6:53–7.

Gadd, S., Kamath, K.R., Silink, M. & Skerritt, J.H. (1992). Co-existence of coeliac disease and insulin-dependent diabetes mellitus in children: screening sera using an ELISA test for gliadin antibody. *Aust. NZ. J. Med.* 22:256–60.

Grefte, J.M.M., Bouman, J.G., Grond, J., Jansen, W. & Kleibeuker, J.H. (1988). Slow and incomplete histological and functional recovery in adult gluten sensitive enteropathy. *J. Clin. Pathol.* 41:886–91.

Holmes, G.K.T. (1989). Malignancy in coeliac disease–effect of a gluten free diet. *Gut* 30:333–8.

Marsh, M.N. (1992). Gluten, major histocompatibility complex and the small intestine. A molecular and immunobiologic approach to the spectrum of gluten sensitivity. *Gastroenterology* 102:330–54.

Penttila, I.A., Gibson, C.E., Forrest, B.D., Cummins, A.G. & LaBrooy, J.T. (1990). Lymphocyte activation as measured by interleukin-2 receptor expression to gluten fraction III in coeliac disease. *Immunol. Cell Biol.* 68:155–60.

Trier, J.S. (1991) Celiac sprue. *N. Engl. J. Med.* 325:1709–19.

12 Inflammatory disorders of the colon

Ian Roberts-Thomson

Introduction

Of several inflammatory disorders of the colon, ulcerative colitis and Crohn's disease are important causes of diarrhoea of moderate or greater severity in developed countries. The clinical manifestations of these disorders in the elderly will be the major focus of this chapter.

Other inflammatory disorders of the colon which can cause diarrhoea, such as ischaemic colitis, diverticulitis, collagenous colitis and pneumatosis coli, will be reviewed briefly since they are predominant in the elderly. Radiation colitis (see Chapter 15), pseudomembraneous colitis (see Chapter 8) and amoebic colitis (see Chapter 8) are discussed elsewhere.

In ulcerative colitis and Crohn's disease, care must be taken with the extrapolation of old data to current clinical outcomes. For example, early data suggested that ulcerative colitis in the elderly often pursued an aggressive course with a poor response to medical therapy and a high perioperative mortality. These observations have not been supported by more recent studies. Reasons for these discrepancies may include nonrecognition of mild forms of inflammatory bowel disease and diagnostic errors in some patients subjected to surgery. For example, the clinical features of Crohn's colitis and ischaemic colitis were only clearly defined in 1960 and 1963, respectively.

Ulcerative colitis and Crohn's disease

Epidemiology

The prevalence of ulcerative colitis and Crohn's disease in various populations, changes in prevalence rates with time and the identification of environmental factors which may predispose to inflammatory bowel disease, have been addressed in various studies. All are compromised to some extent by difficulties with case identification through mortality statistics, hospital admission rates and attendances at outpatient clinics or radiological facilities. Nevertheless, the prevalence of ulcerative colitis is highest in white populations in developed countries, with rates in the region of 50 to 100 per 100000 population. In Europe and the USA, ulcerative colitis may be more common in Jews than in other racial groups. Crohn's disease is also more common in white populations in developed countries, with prevalence rates of about 50 per 100000 population in several areas in the USA and Northern Europe. A study on Crohn's disease within the USA showed that prevalence rates per 100000 for Hispanics (4.1) and Asians (5.6) were much lower than those for whites (43.6) and blacks (29.8). Countries with a low incidence of inflammatory bowel disease include Japan and Eastern Europe and much of Africa, Asia and South America.

Over the past 40 years, the number of new cases of ulcerative colitis per year appears to have been relatively stable in most white populations. In contrast, most studies have shown at least a four-fold increase in the incidence of Crohn's disease. This increase largely occurred in the 1960s and 1970s and may have plateaued in the 1980s. Although environmental factors have been explored, the only consistent associations relate to nonsmoking and ulcerative colitis, and smoking and Crohn's disease. This may reflect the impact of smoking on the nature of inflammatory bowel disease in genetically-susceptible individuals. Weaker associations have been found between Crohn's disease, use of oral contraceptives and a high dietary intake of sugar. Children who are not breast fed may be more likely to develop inflammatory bowel disease but the data is not persuasive.

Most studies have demonstrated a bimodal distribution in the age of onset for both ulcerative colitis and Crohn's disease. This bimodal distribution is unexplained. It has been suggested that the second peak represents an entirely different disease, while others favour a similar disease process, perhaps promoted by physiological changes associated with aging. The possibility that the second peak in later life is related to misclassification of a variety of conditions is no longer tenable.

Women are more frequently affected than men with a female:male ratio of about 1.5:1. In ulcerative colitis, about 12 per cent of patients develop the disease after the age of 60 years and this may be more common in men than women. In Crohn's disease, about 16 per cent are over the age of 60 years – a group which largely consists of women with left-sided Crohn's colitis.

Pathogenesis

Despite considerable research activity, the aetiology of inflammatory bowel disease remains unclear. It is also unclear whether ulcerative colitis and Crohn's disease are separate diseases or different manifestations of similar pathogenic mechanisms. The latter possibility is supported by family studies where some individuals have ulcerative colitis and others have Crohn's disease. In monozygotic twins, concordance is common in Crohn's disease but less common in ulcerative colitis. Some progress has been made with the identification of genetic regions relevant to Crohn's disease but the actual genes and their function remain unclear. Weak associations with HLA antigens have been identified in some populations.

The immunological theories of inflammatory bowel disease can be divided into those which regard the diseases as autoimmune in nature, and those which view the inflammation as an exaggeration or amplification of normal 'physiological' inflammation. Supporters of the autoimmune theory point to associations with other autoimmune disorders, the presence of anticolon antibodies and autoreactive lymphocytes in peripheral blood, and responses to prednisolone and other immunosuppressive drugs. Others have emphasized a variety of immunological changes involving peripheral blood and mucosal lymphocytes, synthesis of immunoglobulin and immune responses to a variety of luminal antigens. In most studies, faecal levels of inflammatory mediators such as leukotrienes and prostaglandins have been higher in ulcerative colitis than in Crohn's disease.

Metabolic theories for the pathogenesis of ulcerative colitis include a deficiency in the ability of gut epithelial cells to metabolize luminal nutrients such as short-chain fatty acids, and impaired degradation or increased synthesis of particular bacterial peptides which stimulate mucosal leucocytes. An additional factor might involve changes in mucus glycoproteins secreted by epithelial cells. In the study of Crohn's disease, there is continuing interest in the possibility of infectious agents, perhaps atypical mycobacteria, viruses, mycoplasmas or bacterial variants with defective cell walls. The permeability of the intestine to various dietary components may also be relevant to Crohn's disease since dietary modification and elemental diets appear to be of some help.

Clinical features

In ulcerative colitis, symptoms are largely determined by the extent and severity of colonic inflammation. The classical triad of abdominal symptoms consists of diarrhoea, rectal bleeding and abdominal pain. Rarely, patients with proctitis may complain of both constipation and the passage of small amounts of blood and mucus. In typical patients, abdominal pain is rarely severe and is usually relieved by defaecation. Systemic symptoms include fever, malaise, anorexia and weight loss. In addition, up to 25 per cent of patients may show remote manifestations including arthritis, aphthous ulceration, iritis, erythema nodosum, pyoderma gangrenosum and a variety of hepatic and biliary disorders.

Several studies have shown a tendency for ulcerative colitis to be less extensive in older than younger patients. For example, one large study showed that the frequency of proctitis in patients over 60 years of age (42 per cent) was higher than that in patients under 60 years (33 per cent). In another study, the mean age for the development of proctitis was about a decade later than that for more extensive disease. Despite this, older patients appear to be more likely to present with a severe initial attack, are more likely to develop a toxic megacolon, and have a higher short-term mortality.

In contrast to ulcerative colitis, the presenting symptoms of Crohn's disease are more variable and include abdominal pain (87 per cent), diarrhoea (66 per cent), weight loss (55 per cent), anorexia (37 per cent) and fever (36 per cent). Malaise, nausea, vomiting and various perianal manifestations, including fissures and fistulas, are also common. The frequency of remote manifestations is similar to that in ulcerative colitis, apart from a higher frequency of oral aphthous ulceration and a lower frequency of hepatobiliary disorders. Physical examination may reveal an abdominal mass, anal skin tags, perianal inflammation and fissures or fistulas.

Several surveys of Crohn's disease have shown a decrease in ileal involvement and an increase in colonic involvement with advancing age. Thus, disease confined to the colon is present in about 60 per cent of patients over the age of 60 compared to 25 per cent of younger patients. At least two-thirds of patients presenting with Crohn's colitis after the age of 60 years are women. In both forms of inflammatory bowel disease, the frequency of extraintestinal manifestations, such as arthritis, appears to be similar in old and young patients.

Investigations and management

In elderly patients, results of investigations for inflammatory bowel disease are similar to those in younger patients. For Crohn's disease, however, delays in diagnosis appear to be more common in the elderly and this may be due, in part, to the more indolent presentation of Crohn's disease involving the distal colon.

Since ulcerative colitis almost always involves the rectum, the diagnosis is usually made by sigmoidoscopy and rectal biopsy. For definition of the extent of the disease, colonoscopy with serial biopsies is usually superior to barium enema x-ray. A detailed description of histological and radiological changes is given in Chapter 5. A typical radiograph in ulcerative colitis is shown in Figure 12.1. In general, patients with more severe disease are more likely to have anaemia, a low plasma albumin and an elevated white cell count, platelet count and ESR. The extent and severity of disease can also be assessed by labelled leucocyte scans and by the faecal excretion of alpha 1-antitrypsin.

The diagnosis of Crohn's disease often depends on the combined impact of clinical, radiological and pathological findings. Ileitis is usually demonstrated by barium follow-through x-ray, while colitis may be shown by colonoscopy or barium enema x-ray (Figure 12.2). If possible, the diagnosis should be supported by histological changes, in part to exclude disorders which may mimic Crohn's disease such as adenocarcinoma, lymphoma or tuberculosis.

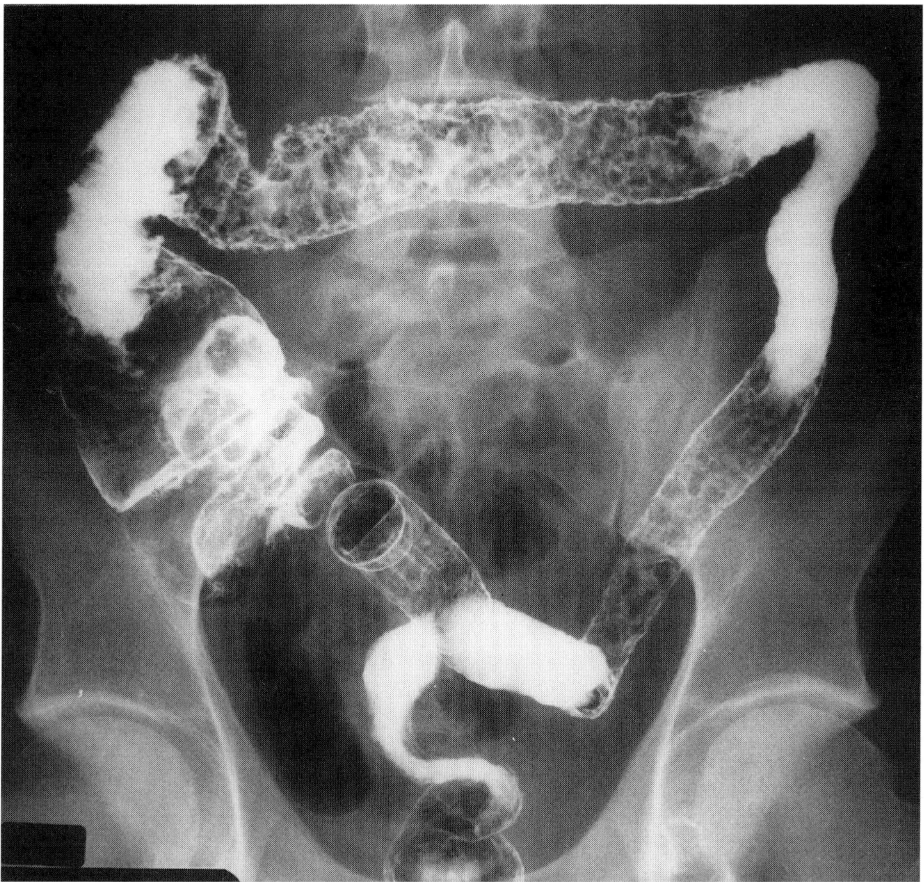

Figure 12.1. Contrast barium enema in active ulcerative colitis showing loss of haustra, a coarse granular mucosa and superficial ulceration, particularly in the transverse colon.

The management of inflammatory bowel disease includes the treatment of acute attacks and the maintenance of remission. In ulcerative colitis, treatment of the acute attack usually requires oral or rectal corticosteroids. Sulfasalazine and related drugs may be helpful but are especially of value in reducing the risk of relapse after induction of remission. In patients with continuing inflammation despite corticosteroids, therapeutic options include the use of immunosuppressive drugs and surgical resection followed by ileostomy or the creation of an ileal pouch.

In Crohn's disease, drug therapy is similar to that in ulcerative colitis but may include the use of metronidazole, particularly for perianal inflammation. In addition, some patients with Crohn's disease respond to semidigested (elemental) diets, although palatability and patient compliance with some preparations is poor. For both forms of inflammatory bowel disease, drug therapy may include symptomatic

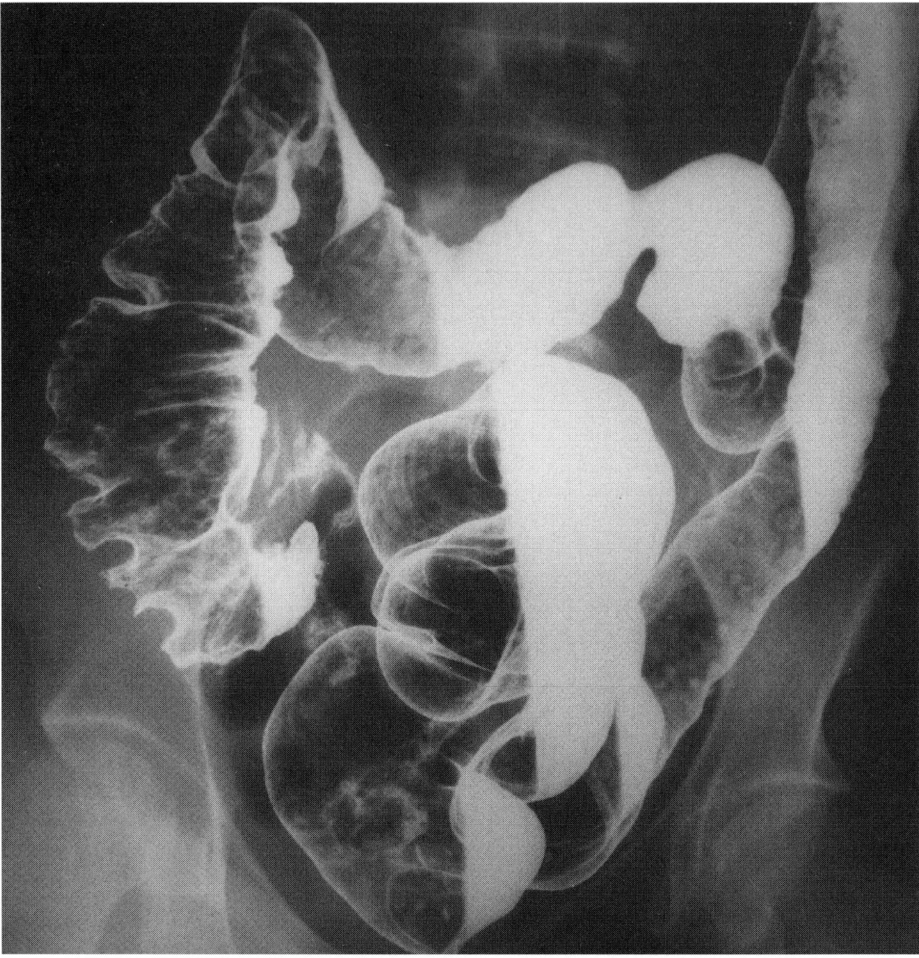

Figure 12.2. Contrast barium enema in Crohn's colitis showing loss of haustra, typical aphthous ulcers in the descending colon and deeper ulcers in the transverse colon.

treatment for pain and diarrhoea and correction of a variety of deficiency states, particularly iron deficiency.

Responses to drug therapy appear to be similar in old and young patients. The observation in one study that elderly patients with Crohn's disease were less likely to receive treatment with either corticosteroids or sulfasalazine probably reflects the higher frequency of milder disease. In ulcerative colitis, the colectomy rate in older patients (8 per cent) was similar to that in younger patients (11 per cent). In Crohn's disease, surgical rates are higher in ileal disease than colonic disease and, because of this, are higher in young than in old patients. Nevertheless, surgical rates in the elderly may reach 30–40 per cent, usually within five years after diagnosis.

Long-term outcome

Recent epidemiological surveys have found that overall survival rates in ulcerative colitis differ only marginally from those of the general population. In Denmark, for example, a slight excess mortality was noted among men over the age of 40 years, but only in the first two years after diagnosis. An additional consideration is the increased risk of development of colon cancer, particularly in patients with pancolitis. This risk increases when the duration of disease exceeds ten years and may reach 20 per cent at 20 years after diagnosis. Although the methods for surveillance are still debated, it is recommended that patients whose duration of disease exceeds 10 years should have a colonoscopy with multiple biopsies every two years.

As noted above, surgical rates in Crohn's disease are lower in elderly patients and reflect the higher frequency of disease confined to the distal colon. After bowel resection, rates for recurrence of disease and rates for further surgery are lower in old than in young patients.

Mortality rates in Crohn's disease are about twice those of the general population and are highest for those who develop the disease under the age of 20 years. Indeed, the risk of death decreases with increasing age at diagnosis and with time from diagnosis. Thus, in at least two studies, older patients with Crohn's disease had a similar mortality to that of the general population.

Ischaemic colitis

Vascular disorders involving the small and large bowel include acute mesenteric ischaemia, chronic mesenteric ischaemia and colonic ischaemia. Acute mesenteric ischaemia mostly presents as a surgical emergency and has a mortality rate of 50–70 per cent. Chronic mesenteric ischaemia is rare and may present with typical mesenteric angina or a variety of symptoms including pain, anorexia, weight loss, constipation and diarrhoea.

Colonic ischaemia is the most common vascular disorder and the only one usually accompanied by diarrhoea. The most common manifestation is 'transient ischaemic colitis' but other syndromes exist including 'chronic ulcerative ischaemic colitis', 'ischaemic colonic stricture' and 'gangrenous ischaemic colitis'.

Ischaemic colitis results from impaired blood flow in the region of the splenic flexure. This is the site of anastomoses between the middle colic artery, which is derived from the superior mesenteric artery, and the left colic artery, which is derived from the inferior mesenteric artery. At least 90 per cent of patients are over 60 years of age and many have evidence of widespread atherosclerosis. Up to 20 per cent of patients may also have potentially obstructing lesions of the colon including carcinomas and strictures associated with diverticulitis.

A typical presentation involves pain of mild to moderate severity, largely in the left abdomen. Subsequently, within hours, bloody diarrhoea or the passage of bright blood per rectum occurs. Patients with more severe pain may experience nausea and vomiting. On examination, patients are not critically ill but may have tachycardia and a mild fever. Abdominal examination reveals tenderness and guarding on the left side of the abdomen. Bowel sounds are usually present. Sigmoidoscopy is normal apart from the presence of blood in the lumen.

In 20 per cent of patients, the diagnosis of ischaemic colitis is supported by a plain abdominal x-ray showing thickening of the large bowel wall by submucosal haemorrhage and oedema. A barium enema x-ray is usually diagnostic but care must be taken to avoid vigorous purgation or overdistension of the colon. Typical features include loss of the haustral pattern, ulceration and marginal filling defects (thumb printing) as shown in Figure 12.3. Colonoscopy may reveal varying degrees of necrosis, inflammation, ulceration and sloughing, which are maximal at five to ten days after the onset of pain.

Treatment with analgesics and intravenous fluids usually results in improvement after two to five days. A repeat barium enema x-ray after two weeks may be appropriate if the diagnosis is in doubt. Radiological changes resolve spontaneously and completely in at least half of the patients while some develop a colonic stricture (20 per cent), chronic ischaemic colitis (10 per cent), and gangrene with perforation (10 per cent). A recurrence of ischaemic colitis occurs in only 5 per cent of patients, while a subsequent episode of acute mesenteric ischaemia is extremely rare. The mortality from ischaemic colitis is low and largely occurs in the small subgroup with gangrene and perforation.

Diverticulitis

Diverticulitis is an inflammatory condition which involves one or more colonic diverticula and is almost always symptomatic.

Diverticula can be found throughout the gastrointestinal tract but are most common in the sigmoid and descending colon. Diverticulosis refers to the presence of one or more diverticula but has no implications with regard to symptoms. Symptomatic diverticular disease refers to diverticulosis associated with symptoms but without evidence of complications such as inflammation.

There is a clear association between diverticulosis and advancing age in western countries. For example, diverticulosis is rare under 30 years of age but increases to occur in more than 50 per cent of the population over 70 years of age. In addition, the number of diverticula per patient also appears to increase with advancing age.

In contrast to western countries, diverticulosis is rare in Asia and Africa, perhaps because of a high intake of dietary fibre. The fibre hypothesis is supported by results

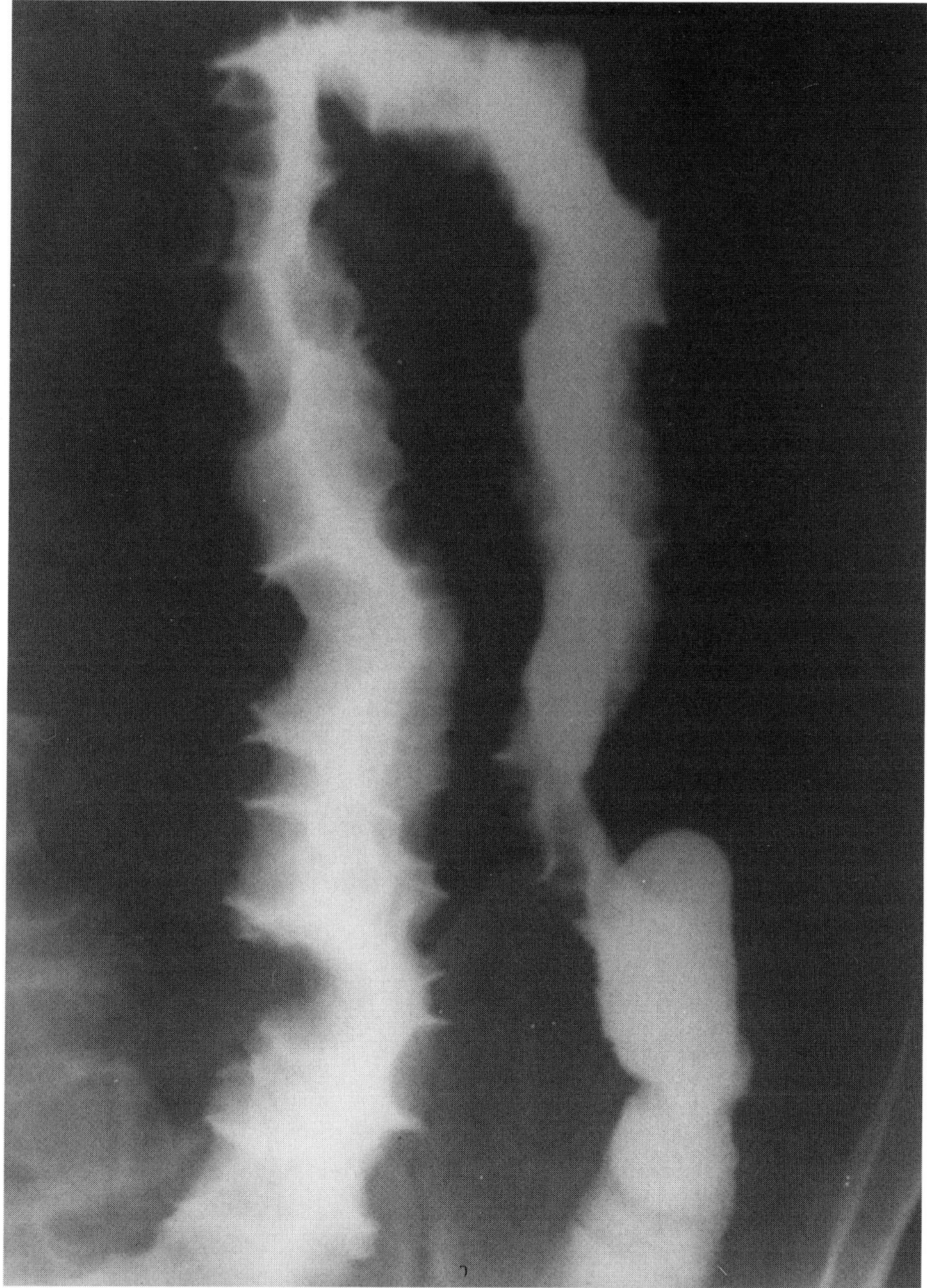

Figure 12.3. Barium enema in ischaemic colitis showing typical marginal filling defects (thumb printing) around the splenic flexure.

from dietary surveys and by the finding of a lower prevalence of diverticular disease in vegetarians than in nonvegetarians. Although the pathogenesis is still debated, diverticulosis may result from the combined effects of a low faecal mass, hypertrophy of circular smooth muscle and the subsequent generation of high intraluminal pressures.

At least 80 per cent of patients with diverticulosis are either completely asymptomatic or have only minor symptoms which are insufficient to lead to medical consultation. Of the remainder, three-quarters have painful diverticular disease while one-quarter develop either diverticulitis or haemorrhage.

Diverticulitis may develop in about 5 per cent of patients with diverticulosis. The most common mechanism is now thought to be a small perforation which occurs during episodes of raised intracolonic pressure. Alternatively, inspissated faecal material may lodge in the orifice of the diverticulum, resulting in inflammation and perforation. The most common outcome is a pericolic abscess which occasionally results in fistulas to the bladder, vagina, skin or small bowel. Free perforation into the peritoneal cavity is rare and usually presents as a surgical emergency. Pericolic abscesses have a variable natural history and may enlarge with worsening symptoms or resolve by repair processes or spontaneous drainage back into the colonic lumen.

The major symptoms are those of abdominal pain and a change in bowel habit. Pain is usually abrupt in onset and is typically localized to the lower abdomen, particularly the left iliac fossa. A change in bowel habit is noted by 40–50 per cent of patients and takes the form of persisting constipation, intermittent constipation or intermittent diarrhoea. Additional symptoms may include nausea, vomiting, fever and urinary symptoms. Physical examination usually reveals tenderness in the left lower quadrant and there may be an abdominal mass if the abscess is relatively large.

Laboratory investigations show a leucocytosis and a raised erythrocyte sedimentation rate (ESR). The urinary sediment may reveal an excess of red or white blood cells when the urinary tract is involved in the inflammatory process. Sigmoidoscopy should be performed early to exclude cancer and inflammatory bowel disease involving the rectum. Plain abdominal radiographs may show a degree of dilatation of the large bowel consistent with either an ileus or partial obstruction. A barium enema x-ray is normally delayed for one month and may reveal changes as in Figure 12.4. Some patients will need additional investigations including colonoscopy, ultrasound and CT scans.

Most patients with diverticulitis require hospitalization, analgesics, intravenous therapy and parenteral antibiotics. Typical antibiotic regimens involve triple therapy with ampicillin, gentamicin and metronidazole or a newer cephalosporin combined with metronidazole. At least 70 per cent of patients improve in

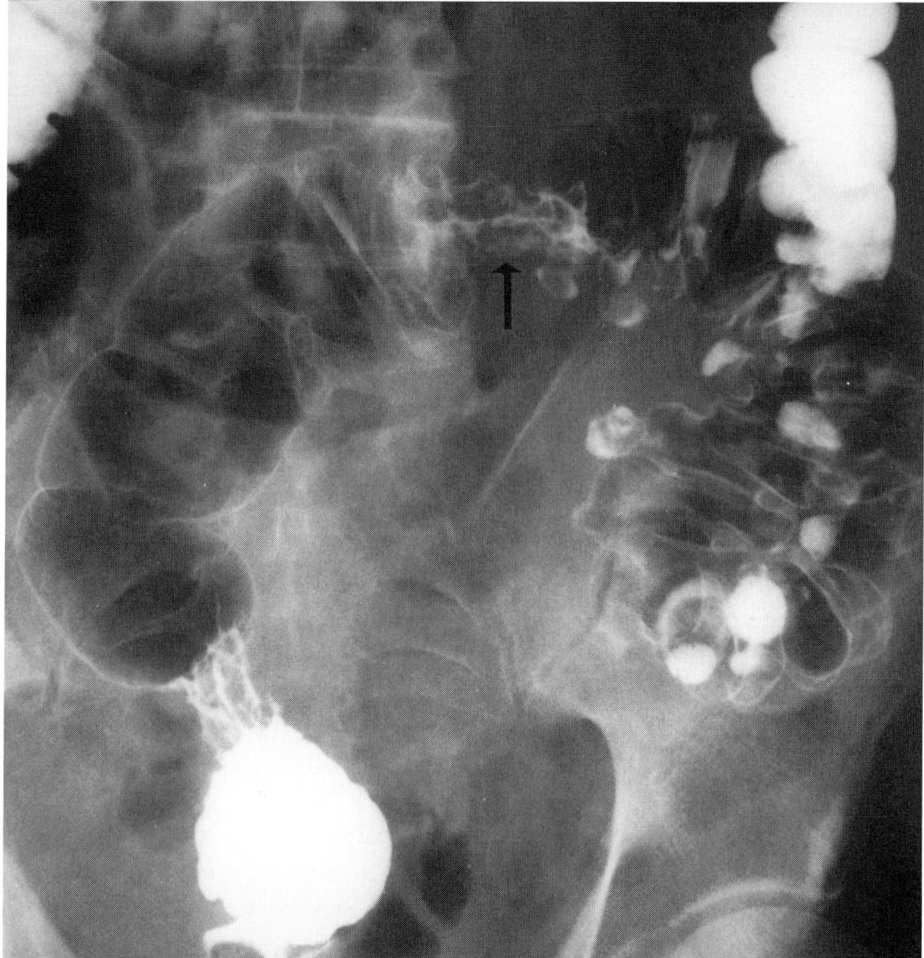

Figure 12.4. Contrast barium enema in a patient with diverticulosis and previous diverticulitis showing a stricture in the lower sigmoid colon (arrow).

3–7 days, after which patients can resume a normal diet before discharge from hospital.

About 5 per cent of patients treated conservatively may subsequently require surgery for complications such as abscess formation, fistulas, strictures and persisting inflammation. Diverticulitis recurs in about 25 per cent of patients, usually within five years of the initial attack.

The classical features of diverticulitis may be less prominent in patients over 80 years of age and in those with coexisting disorders such as dementia. In such patients, a high index of suspicion is required to avoid potential problems associated with delays in diagnosis and treatment.

Collagenous colitis

Collagenous colitis is a rare disorder characterized by diarrhoea, a normal or near-normal colon at endoscopy and by characteristic changes in colonic biopsies including thickening of the collagen band beneath the surface epithelium. Patients with this disorder have a mean age of 55–60 years of age and are four times more likely to be women than men.

At presentation, the major symptom is watery diarrhoea which may be intermittent or persistent and has usually been present for months or years. Additional symptoms may include abdominal cramps, nausea, vomiting and weight loss. Barium enema x-rays are normal while colonoscopy reveals either a normal mucosa or only mild colonic oedema.

Laboratory investigations may reveal an elevated ESR and a mild eosinophilia. The histological hallmark is excessive deposition of collagen (type III) below the surface epithelium. This may range in thickness from 7 to 100 μm (compared with normal values of 1 to 7 μm), and may vary in different parts of the colon. There is always an increase in chronic inflammatory cells in the lamina propria (lymphocytes, plasma cells and eosinophils) and sometimes an increase in mucosal neutrophils (Figure 12.5). Subepithelial fibrosis is likely to be due to the chronic inflammatory process but another explanation is a local abnormality of collagen synthesis. The mechanism of diarrhoea, although debated, may involve a reduction in the capacity of the colon to absorb fluid and electrolytes. Jejunal perfusion studies suggest impaired small bowel absorption in some patients.

Treatment consists of nonspecific constipating agents such as loperamide and codeine phosphate. Symptoms resolve spontaneously in some patients while others respond to treatment with bismuth subsalicylate or perhaps to sulfasalazine, corticosteroids or mepacrine.

Microscopic colitis

Microscopic colitis has similar clinical and histological features to collagenous colitis but colonic inflammation is not associated with subepithelial fibrosis. A consensus view is that microscopic colitis and collagenous colitis are related diseases, perhaps different stages in the evolution of a single inflammatory process.

Pneumatosis coli

Pneumatosis coli is another rare disorder characterized by the presence of gas-filled cysts in the subserosa or submucosa. The cysts probably result from gas production

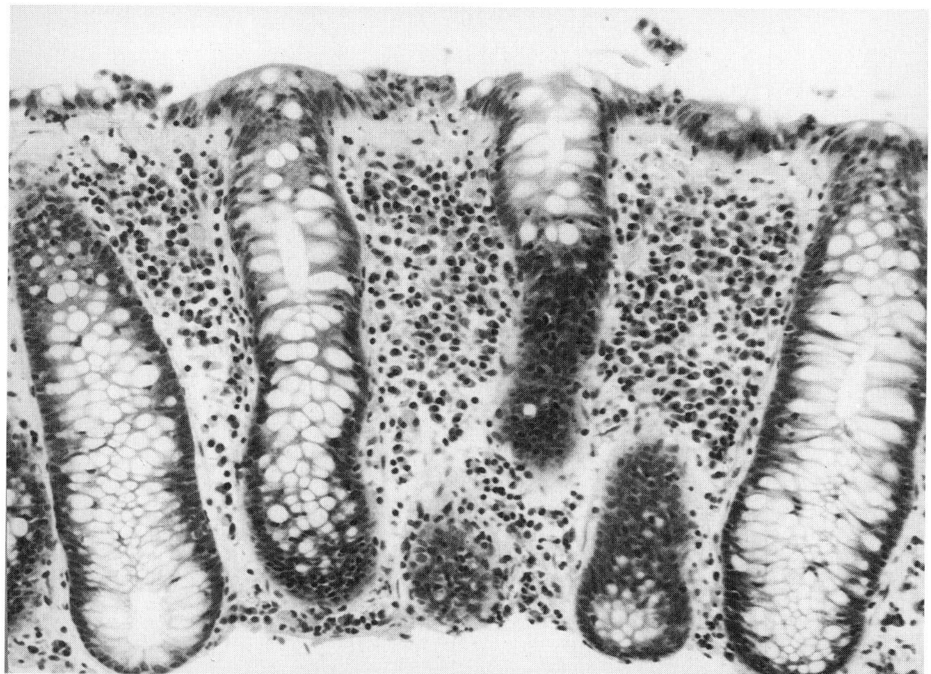

Figure 12.5. Microscopic appearance of collagenous colitis showing an increase in inflammatory cells in the lamina propria, changes in surface epithelial cells and a thick band of collagen beneath the surface epithelium. (Kindly supplied by Dr R Whitehead, Adelaide.)

by enteric bacteria in the colonic wall, but other explanations include tracking of air from a ruptured alveolus in the lung through the mediastinum and intestinal mesentery.

Patients are almost always elderly and some have coexisting disorders such as chronic airways limitation or colonic inflammation due to diverticulitis or pseudo-membranous colitis. The disease appears to be more common in men than in women and may be asymptomatic or cause mild diarrhoea, sometimes with blood and mucus in stools. If the rectum is involved, sigmoidoscopy is abnormal with submucosal blebs, often associated with features of mild inflammation.

The disorder may be recognized on a plain abdominal radiograph but a barium enema x-ray is diagnostic (Figure 12.6). If patients are symptomatic, improvement almost always occurs after hospitalization and the administration of 70 per cent oxygen by mask for five days. Variable responses have been reported with antibiotics, sulfasalazine and elemental diets. Unfortunately, after successful therapy, the majority of patients relapse within 12 months.

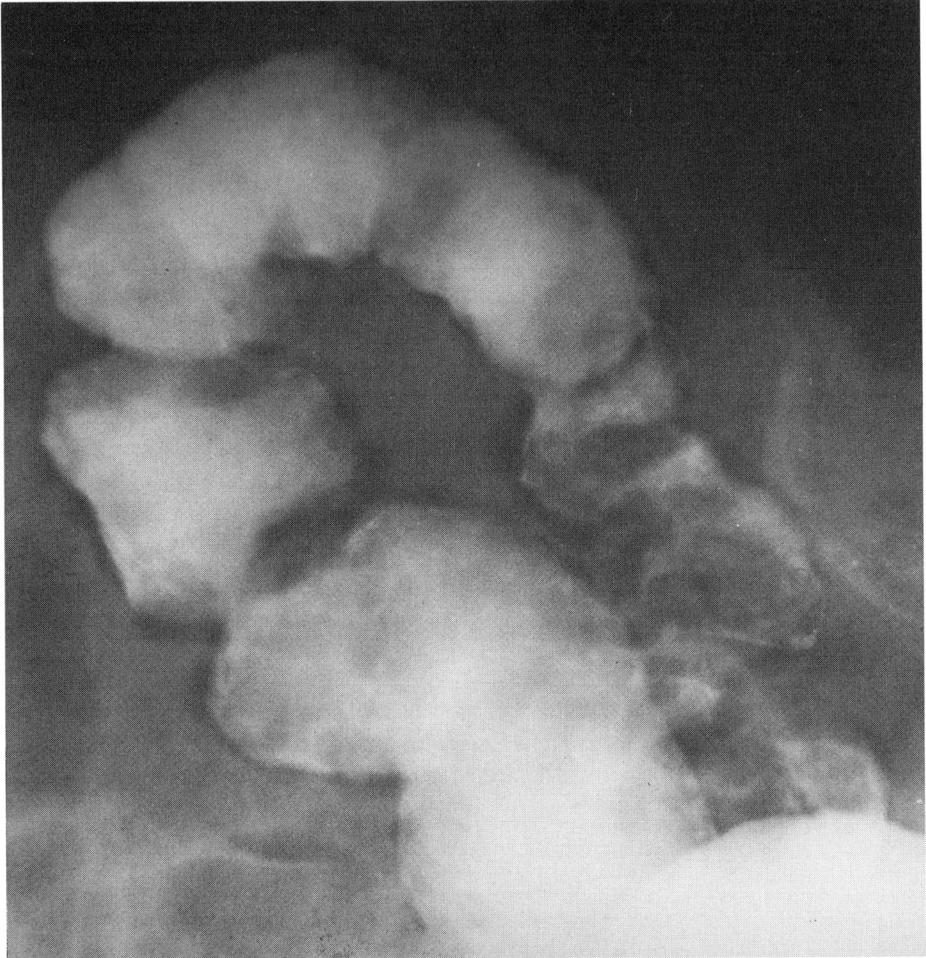

Figure 12.6. Barium enema in pneumatosis coli showing gas-containing cysts in the wall of the rectum and sigmoid colon and distortion of the sigmoid lumen.

BIBLIOGRAPHY AND FURTHER READING

Brandt, L.J., Boley, S.J. & Mitsudo, S. (1982). Clinical characteristics and natural history of colitis in the elderly. *Am. J. Gastroenterol* 77:382–6.

Courtney, M.G., Nunes, D.P., Bergin, C.F. et al. (1992). Randomised comparison of olsalazine and mesalazine in prevention of relapses in ulcerative colitis. *Lancet* **339**:1279–81.

Grimm, I. & Friedman, S. (1990). Inflammatory bowel disease in the elderly. *Gastroenterol. Clin. North Am.* **19**:361–89.

Misiewicz, J.J. & Pounder, R.E. (eds.) (1987). *Diseases of the Gut and Pancreas.* Oxford: Blackwell.

Myren, J., Bouchier, I.A., Watkinson, G., Softley, A., Clamp, S.E. & de Dombal, F.T. (1988). The

OMGE multinational inflammatory bowel disease survey 1976–1986. A further report on 3175 cases. *Scand. J. Gastroenterol. Suppl.* **144**:11–9.

Peppercorn, M.A. (1990). Advances in drug therapy for inflammatory bowel disease. *Ann. Intern. Med.* **112**:50–60.

Podolsky, D.K. (1991). Inflammatory bowel disease. I. *N. Engl. J. Med.* **325**:928–37.

Podolsky, D.K. (1991). Inflammatory bowel disease. II. *N. Engl. J. Med.* **325**:1008–16.

Rams, H., Rogers, A.I. & Ghandur-Mnaymneh, L. (1987). Collagenous colitis. *Ann. Intern. Med.* **106**:108–13.

Ruderman, W.B. (1990). Newer pharmacologic agents for the therapy of inflammatory bowel disease. *Med. Clin. North Am.* **74**:133–53.

Shearman, D.J.C. & Finlayson N.D.C. (eds.) (1989). *Diseases of the Gastrointestinal Tract and Liver.* Edinburgh: Churchill Livingstone

Sleisenger, M.H. & Fordtran, J.S. (eds.) (1989). *Gastrointestinal Disease: Pathophysiology, Diagnosis, Management,* 4th edn, Vol. 2. Philadelphia: Saunders.

Whelan, G. (1990). Epidemiology of inflammatory bowel disease. *Med. Clin. North Am.* **74**:1–12.

13 Neoplasia and diarrhoea

James McA. Cooper

Introduction

The gastrointestinal tract is one of the most common sites of tumour. The malignancies of the lower gastrointestinal tract, predominantly carcinoma of the colon and of the rectum, are responsible for one in eight of all deaths from cancer. This is exceeded only by carcinomas of the lung. In the USA approximately 160 000 new cancers of the lower gastrointestinal tract will be diagnosed each year.

Tumours arise in populations of dividing cells. They are clonal and arise secondary to a single or multiple genetic mutation in a dividing cell. It is at cell division, when the cell's DNA is being copied, that permanent changes in the genome of that cell will occur. Populations of cells, therefore, such as those at the epithelial surfaces of the colon and lung, and hematopoietic cells, where the proliferation of cells is active, are prone to the development of cancer.

Adenocarcinomas are responsible for most of the morbidity and mortality associated with tumours of the gastrointestinal tract. Other neoplasia such as the tubular adenomas are extremely common and seldom of consequence. Adenomatous polyps are now recognized as having potential for malignant transformation. Up to 10 per cent of all colorectal cancer can be related to primary inherited genetic abnormalities while up to 70 per cent of all colorectal cancers will have predisposing genetic factors.

Tumours of the gastrointestinal tract may present late due to a lack of specific symptoms. Anaemia, fatigue and weight loss are common. Tumours of the large bowel may in addition present with obvious blood loss but a large percentage will present with alteration of bowel habit. In some series of carcinoma and villous adenoma of the colon and rectum, up to 60 per cent of patients complain of diarrhoea. Mucus secretion by villous adenomas may be extreme but colorectal carcinoma presents as diarrhoea much more commonly than is recognized.

Tumours of the small bowel may present with obstruction or with symptoms due to the secretion of excessive hormones (see Chapter 15).

154

Pathology of intestinal tumours

Less than 1 per cent of all gastrointestinal malignancies occur in the small intestine. Of these, 50 per cent are adenocarcinomas and 75 per cent of these involve the ampulla of Vater. Carcinoid tumours, lymphoma and leiomyosarcomas account for the bulk of the remainder. Within the large intestine, adenocarcinoma is the most important lesion and the relationship of these malignancies to nonmalignant adenomatous lesions is now well established. However, a variety of polyps that lack malignant potential may also occur in the colon. The most common are the hyperplastic polyp and inflammatory polyp. Hamartomatous polyps, such as those occurring in Peutz–Jeghers syndrome, seem not to have intrinsic transforming capacity. However, the higher incidence of gastrointestinal tumours, especially of the stomach and duodenum, in this syndrome suggests an underlying predisposition to tumour formation.

Adenoma

Of great importance in terms of the development of malignancies in the colon are the premalignant adenomas. Adenomas may be classified histologically as tubular, tubulovillous or villous. Of all adenomas of the bowel, 70 per cent will be tubular, 20 per cent tubulovillous and 10 per cent villous.

Tubular adenomas are present in over 50 per cent of all autopsies. Predominantly they occur in the large bowel. Only 0.05 per cent of these adenomas occur in the small intestine and these may present with obstruction or intussusception. Of those in the large intestine, 20 per cent occur in the caecum, 20 per cent in the ascending or transverse colon, 20 per cent in the sigmoid colon and 20 per cent in the rectum. Generally symptom-free, 50 per cent demonstrate epithelial atypia and occasionally true 'carcinoma in situ' is found. Transformation may occur but with a lower frequency than in villous adenomas. Of lesions greater than 2 cm, transformation occurs in 10 per cent. Less than 1 per cent of those lesions smaller than 1 cm will show transformation. Tubulovillous adenomas, representing some 20 per cent of colonic adenomas, show similar behaviour to tubular adenomas.

Villous adenomas represent only about 5 per cent of colonic adenomas and are most common in the rectum and sigmoid colon. When detected, they are usually greater than 4 cm and more commonly show areas of dysplasia or carcinoma. In lesions greater than 2 cm, up to 40 per cent may show foci of carcinoma. Villous adenomas often present with diarrhoea. Indeed, secretion of up to 3–4 litres of mucus per day may occur.

In all of these adenomas, the likelihood of malignant transformation is related directly to the size of the lesion.

Carcinoma

Carcinoma of the large bowel is very common, with 160 000 new cases each year in the USA. Fifteen per cent of all malignant tumours arise in the colon. Of these, 45 per cent occur in the rectum and, epidemiologically and pathologically, represent a separate entity. While the USA, northern Europe and Australia have similar rates of incidence of these cancers, southern Europe and Japan have a 50 per cent lower incidence. Areas of Africa, Asia and South America have an even lower incidence.

The development of adenocarcinoma is a multistep process. It is now apparent that adenocarcinomas arise in pre-existing adenomatous polyps. Individuals with high numbers of intestinal polyps are therefore at high risk. The likelihood of carcinoma developing in an individual polyp is related to the size of that polyp. Individuals may inherit a predisposition to the development of multiple intestinal polyps in the hereditary polyposis syndromes.

However, other individuals will show an inherited predisposition to colorectal carcinoma that is not associated with an increased number of polyps. These inherited conditions have been named the Lynch syndromes. In these syndromes an increased predisposition to colorectal carcinoma can be identified within the family of the patient with a site predisposition (often for the proximal colon), no increased number of colonic polyps, and a tendency for the cancers to be mucinous and poorly differentiated. In addition, colonic cancers may occur without (Lynch I) or with (Lynch II) an associated increase in risk for extracolonic cancers.

Several genetic loci may be involved in the development of colorectal carcinoma and sequential genetic events are required for development of fully malignant colorectal carcinoma.

Genetics of cancer

The study of cancer has developed greatly in the last 20 years in parallel with the advances being made in molecular biology. It has been known for many years that tumours are clonal. Even the largest tumours arise because of abnormalities in a single initial cell. The progeny of that cell inherit the abnormality which must therefore of necessity be genetic.

It is now clear that the development of a highly malignant, rapidly dividing cancer requires several independent mutations in the genes of the cancer cells. Some individuals inherit an abnormality in their genome from their parents and are thus more susceptible than others to the development of cancer. Hence, both somatic and germline mutations may contribute to oncogenesis.

Tumour cells divide inappropriately. Consequent to this, they tend to show impaired differentiation. These characteristics seem to be inextricably linked.

There are, however, many more steps in tumorigenesis than proliferation. To be malignant, a cell must be able to invade lymphatics or blood vessels, to lodge in distant tissues and to survive in tissues of quite different characteristics from its original organ. A cell that is able to migrate from the wall of the gut and then survive in the lung as a metastasis has achieved much more than simple proliferation.

Abnormal cell proliferation can occur due to two reasons. The cell could respond to increased growth signals. All cells rely on a complex interaction of growth factors (cytokines) that promote proliferation and control organogenesis. One can imagine that an excess of such cytokines or an enhanced response to these cytokines could lead a cell to proliferate abnormally.

Alternatively, cells can be regarded as being under the control of negative, down-regulating signals that may, for example, encourage differentiation in a cell and hence decrease its proliferation. Thus a cell may start proliferating if such negative regulators are destroyed or the cell loses its responsiveness to them.

Both possibilities have received great attention over the last decade. Knowledge of the relevant growth factors has increased greatly and, with respect to cancer, the genes involved in these pathways are known as oncogenes. Conversely, the regulating genes are generally described as tumour suppressor genes (the term 'antioncogene' is misleading).

Genetic mutations in colorectal cancer

Oncogenes are normal genes that exist in all our cells and are critical in normal development. The term 'proto-oncogene' has been coined to describe the normal gene that can mutate to become oncogenic. The genes encode proteins that act either as growth factors, as growth factor receptors, as components of the intracellular signalling pathways or as nucleoproteins that directly influence events within the nucleus. A large number of different oncogenes are responsible for the mitogenic signals that are passed from one cell to another that lead to cell proliferation.

In tumour cells, it is common to find that the normal oncogenes have become mutated or otherwise genetically altered to be overactive or to produce abnormal gene products, i.e. abnormally active growth factors. Up to 50 per cent of all colon and lung carcinomas show mutations within the *ras* oncogene. The *ras* protein is critical to intracellular pathways of mitogenesis. *Ras* mutations are found, for example, in over 90 per cent of pancreatic carcinomas. Abnormal oncogenes can be introduced experimentally into nontumorigenic cells and promote tumour formation. Indeed many oncogenes have been first identified by this means.

It has long been recognized that most cancers are associated with chromosomal deletions and particular cancers show characteristic deletions. Such deletions are often the hallmark of tumour suppressor genes. Colorectal carcinomas show chromosomal deletions or allelic loss at loci on chromosomes 5q, 13q, 17q and 18q. The investigations of these deletions have identified several genetic loci important in the development of these cancers. In addition to activation of the oncogene *ras*, deletions and mutations occur at four loci identified so far: p53, MCC (mutated in colorectal carcinoma), APC (adenomatous polyposis coli) and DCC (deleted in colorectal carcinoma), all of which appear to behave as tumour suppressor genes.

The deletion of DCC, located on chromosome 18q, appears to be a late event in the progression of colorectal carcinoma. It encodes a molecule of homology to the neural cell adhesion molecules (N-CAMs).

While the preceding discussion highlights the importance of the uncontrolled proliferation of cancer cells, one of the most important steps in the development of malignancy is the ability to invade and to metastasize. The observation that loss of a cell adhesion molecule is important in the progression of a cancer is extremely interesting. Such cell adhesion molecules are important for the normal contacts between cells. Cell–cell signalling may be critical in the control of proliferation and also responsible for the interactions between cell and substrate. This may determine the invasive and metastatic potential of cancer cells.

Models of colorectal carcinoma emphasize the importance of this multistep progression from normal epithelium, through adenomatous polyp to carcinoma. A single genetic event will not explain this progression.

In familial adenomatous polyposis coli, one abnormal copy of APC is inherited from the affected parent and one normal copy from the unaffected parent. The normal APC locus is not mutated in adenomatous polyps or cancers. A second event at another genetic locus has therefore occurred in these polyps. By contrast, it is not clear at all that genetic events are required at each of the known loci. Events at one or two of these loci may be sufficient or other loci altogether may be involved. While some of the genetic events appear to occur early in the progress of oncogenesis, the exact sequence is not known.

The ability to screen individuals in affected families for mutations in APC, for example, may provide an early, safe and powerful diagnostic tool.

Clinical presentation

Colorectal carcinoma and other tumours of the gastrointestinal tract are significant causes of morbidity and mortality. Symptoms referable to the gastrointestinal tract occur in some patients with these cancers and many others present with nonspecific symptoms. The diagnosis of these cancers is confounded by the frequency of gastrointestinal symptoms in the general population.

Classically, some distinction has been made between the clinical presentation of carcinoma of the colon arising in the caecum and the right side of the colon, from those of the left side. Bleeding occurs in up to 60 per cent of rectal cancers and 50 per cent of cancers of the splenic flexure and descending colon. By contrast, bleeding is evident in only 5 per cent of lesions in the right side of the colon and the slow loss of blood from these lesions often results in iron deficiency anaemia before any overt bleeding is noticed.

A palpable mass may be felt at presentation in 50 per cent of cases of right-sided cancers while only 10 per cent of left-sided lesions will be palpable, although a high percentage of the left-sided tumours (90 per cent) will be detectable by rectal examination or sigmoidoscopy.

Alteration of bowel habit is an extremely common symptom in all cancers. Diarrhoea, constipation and bowel obstruction may occur depending on the site and pathological characteristics of the tumour. Some studies have estimated that 20 per cent of cancers of the ascending colon present with constipation or diarrhoea, compared with 40 per cent of cancers of the transverse colon. Up to 60 per cent of lesions of the rectum produce some constipation. However, these estimates are conservative compared with other studies that have shown higher rates, particularly of diarrhoea.

In a study of presenting symptoms of carcinoma of the colon, change of bowel habit was the most common symptom at presentation (56 per cent), followed by rectal bleeding (44 per cent), abdominal pain (41 per cent), weight loss (17 per cent), anaemia (11 per cent) and tenesmus (7 per cent).

The common presenting symptoms associated with carcinoma of the colon have generated many attempts to rationalize selection of patients for further investigation. Routine screening of individuals with a strong family history of carcinoma of the colon (three or more first degree relatives) by radiology or flexible sigmoidoscopy is advised. Routine screening of patients with an average risk of carcinoma of the colon, including annual rectal digital examination and occult blood testing annually from the age of 40 years, is recommended by the American Cancer Society. Flexible sigmoidoscopy from the age of 50 years on a 3–5 year basis is also advocated.

However, in other individuals with abdominal symptoms, identification of those for follow-up may be extremely difficult and delays in investigation are common. Within the context of a discussion of diarrhoea in the elderly, a very common complaint in this group of individuals, the decision to investigate is never clear cut.

Diarrhoea and colonic cancer

While there would be little doubt that patients presenting with symptoms of dark or bright red blood loss per rectum require further investigation, what of the patient presenting with unexplained diarrhoea?

The problem has been addressed in several studies, all of which illustrate the clinical problem. In a general, unselected population, 2–4 per cent of individuals will report an episode of diarrhoea within the last two weeks. Diarrhoea generally appears to be a consequence of either excessive secretion of mucus or exudation following local destruction of the normal epithelium with shedding of cells, debris, protein loss and bleeding. Diarrhoea may also be a feature of obstructive lesions, either intermittently or as spurious diarrhoea.

In a survey of 1533 patients, symptoms of bleeding per rectum were noted in 6.6 per cent of patients over a six-month period, diarrhoea in 8.7 per cent and a change in bowel habit in 12.3 per cent. Only one of these individuals had an adenoma present at endoscopy.

However, diarrhoea is nearly as useful a predictor as other symptoms. The predictive value of Hemoccult testing is reported to be 21 per cent, self-reported dark bleeding 16 per cent and diarrhoea 17 per cent. The combination of a positive Hemoccult test in a patient with symptoms increases the predictive value to 46 per cent (and to 57 per cent if the symptom was of dark bleeding per rectum).

In considering patients with proven carcinoma, diarrhoea is a common symptom and up to 60 per cent of patients in some series have presented with diarrhoea alone or together with other symptoms.

Several extracolonic neoplasms cause diarrhoea due to the secretion of excessive hormones by the tumour. These entities are discussed in Chapter 15.

Although unexplained diarrhoea must therefore be taken extremely seriously in the elderly patient, as an isolated symptom the number of colonic tumours discovered on further investigation of diarrhoea will be small and no clear-cut paradigm for investigation exists.

Management and prognosis

It is believed that early recognition of cancers improves the outcome. Direct evidence for this belief is tenuous in carcinoma of the colon and appears to be based on the benefit of early surgical intervention in the hereditary syndromes and on the relationship between staging at diagnosis and prognosis. Using the Duke classification, the five-year survival is directly related to the extent and possibly, but not certainly, to the length of time the tumour has been present. The five-year survival following resection for Duke's A tumours (those restricted to the bowel wall) is above 80 per cent, for Duke's B (with penetration of the bowel wall) 70 per cent, for Duke's C (with lymph node metastasis) 30 per cent and for Duke's D (with distant metastases) only 6 per cent.

Management remains essentially surgical but several developments in the adjuvant chemotherapy of these tumours have taken place. While 5-fluorouracil was shown to have some activity against carcinoma of the colon, it has not been greatly successful as a single agent. The drug has been used in several trials in combination with either levamisole or interferon alpha-2a, and improvement in survival has been demonstrated. Levamisole combined with 5-fluorouracil produces a significant reduction in the incidence of recurrence and the rate of death when used as adjuvant therapy. It seems likely, therefore, that adjuvant therapy will have an increasingly important role in the treatment of these cancers.

Carcinoma of the colon and rectum remains one of the most important malignant tumours. Early recognition provides hope of surgical control. Bleeding, diarrhoea and other alteration of bowel habit must therefore be investigated to make a diagnosis as early as possible.

The genetics of colorectal carcinoma has demonstrated the great importance of tumour suppressor genes. Inherited abnormalities in tumour suppressor genes, such as APC, and acquired mutations in other genes (p 53, DCC and MCC) have been demonstrated in addition to the well recognized activation of oncogenes of the *ras* family. An understanding of these genetic abnormalities has already provided the means to screen families at risk.

BIBLIOGRAPHY AND FURTHER READING

Burt, R.W. & Samowitz, W.S. (1988). The adenomatous polyp and the hereditary polyposis syndromes. *Gastroenterol. Clin. North Am.* 17:657–78.

Farrands, P.A. & Hardcastle, J.D. (1984). Colorectal screening by a self-completion questionnaire. *Gut* 25:445–7.

Kohn, G.J. & Lawson, M.J. (1992). Colorectal cancer. Identifying and screening high-risk patients. *Postgrad. Med.* 91:241–4, 247–53.

Kyle, S.M., Isbister, W.H. & Yeong, M.L. (1991). Presentation, duration of symptoms and staging of colorectal carcinoma. *Aust. NZ. J. Surg.* 61:137–40.

Lynch, H.T., Lanspa, S.J., Boman, B.M. et al. (1988). Hereditary nonpolyposis colorectal cancer – Lynch syndromes I and II. *Gastroenterol. Clin. North Am.* 17:679–712.

Silman, A.J., Mitchell, P., Nicholls, R.J. et al. (1983). Self-reported dark red bleeding as a marker comparable with occult blood testing in screening for large bowel neoplasms. *Br. J. Surg.* 70:721–4.

Solomon, E., Borrow, J. & Goddard, A.D. (1991). Chromosome aberrations and cancer. *Science* 254:1153–60.

Weinberg, R.A. (1991). Tumour suppressor genes. *Science* 254:1138–46.

Young, G.P., Rozen, P. & Levin, B. (eds.) (1996). *Prevention and Early Detection of Colorectal Cancer.* London: Saunders.

14   Irritable bowel syndrome

William M.H. Goh and Ranjit N. Ratnaike

Irritable bowel syndrome (IBS) is probably the most common cause of gastrointestinal dysfunction in the elderly. IBS is considered a benign, noninflammatory, nonprogressive and chronic bowel disorder with numerous symptoms. Over the years this syndrome has been referred to by synonyms such as spastic colon, mucus colitis, nervous diarrhoea and neurotic bowel.

IBS is defined as at least bi-weekly nonmenstrual abdominal distress with diarrhoea, constipation, or alternation between the two, over at least three months, for which no organic cause can be found. Another, more comprehensive, definition is that IBS is 'chronic or recurrent symptoms attributable to the intestines and occurring in varying but characteristic combinations of abdominal pain, bloatedness (distension) and symptoms of disordered defaecation, especially urgency, straining, feeling of incomplete evacuation and altered stool form and frequency'.

There is no data to suggest that the symptoms of IBS in the elderly are different from younger patients. Although much has been written about IBS, information on people over the age of 65 years is limited.

In a survey of 328 subjects over the age of 65 years by Talley and colleagues (1992) the prevalence of symptoms compatible with IBS was 10.9 per 100.

Epidemiology

Irrespective of age, at least half the patients who complain of gastrointestinal symptoms are diagnosed as suffering from IBS. About five million people within the European Community are likely to have IBS. The cost incurred in diagnosis and treatment of these patients is around $300–600 per patient.

The age distribution of patients with IBS does not show a preponderance in the elderly age group. In a series of 320 patients from the Mayo Clinic, 16 per cent of the patients were over the age of 56 years. Regarding gender, IBS is more common in females and in most large series the female:male ratio is 2:1.

The epidemiology of IBS is likely to change with time as the definition of the condition becomes more precise and a diagnostic test is available.

Pathogenesis

Despite many hypotheses on the cause of IBS there is no unanimity nor a specific organic explanation. The factors associated with IBS include: an increase in contractibility of the bowel; chronic excessive parasympathetic stimulation of the bowel; idiosyncratic response to cholecystokinin and pentagastrin; variations in intraluminal pressure; and fibre deficiency and neurotransmitter substances in bowel tissues. In the elderly, physiological changes in the aging gut could theoretically be significant in the aetiology of IBS.

Clinicians taking a comprehensive history from IBS patients often elicit the occurrence of stress at the onset of symptoms. It is reported that 75 per cent of patients have a psychological factor which may be related to the onset or exacerbation of the condition. The relationship between psychosocial stressors and IBS remains controversial. There is considerable variation in how individuals perceive normal life events as stressful. IBS patients rate more stressors in their lives compared to control groups and possibly perceive life as more stressful.

Some studies reveal that IBS patients tend to function at a higher level of anxiety and, compared with control groups, have higher autonomic arousal. Individuals experience and express their distress in different ways cognitively, affectively and physiologically. IBS patients are probably predisposed to respond to stress with gut symptoms. Individuals who perceive normal life events as more stressful, who begin life with a higher autonomic arousal and express stress with intestinal symptoms, may develop IBS.

A possible mechanism between perception of a psychosocial stressor and IBS is as follows:

Stressor → Perceived threat → Autonomic arousal → Gut symptom → IBS

Elderly people are more preoccupied with their bowel habits than younger persons, to whom sexual functions are more important. Obsessional individuals often elaborate on their bowel habits and rituals. In patients with IBS, traits of orderliness, cleanliness, punctuality and inflexibility are often noticed by clinicians. It is currently held, however, that no specific personality patterns are associated with these patients.

Studies have revealed that about 25 per cent of IBS patients have a psychiatric disorder such as dysthymic disorder, unipolar depression or an attention deficit disorder. These findings are of particular relevance to the elderly, who are more likely to suffer from anxiety and depression due to altered circumstances such as bereavement of a spouse, ill health, a lack of a life purpose, loneliness, institutionalization and perhaps introspection regarding death.

Symptoms

The variety of symptoms experienced by patients with IBS are listed below.

Pain
- Abdominal distress
- Excruciating pain
- Cramping
- Burning.

Erratic bowel action
- Diarrhoea
- Constipation
- Watery stools
- Stringy stools
- Mucus stools.

Gaseousness
- Flatulence
- Fullness
- Pressure.

Other symptoms
- Headaches
- Giddiness
- Urinary frequency
- Fatigue
- Lassitude
- Shortness of breath.

In one large series, 70 per cent of patients with IBS complained of the symptom triad of abdominal pain, altered bowel habit and flatulence; only 10 per cent of 209 patients with organic disease have similar complaints.

Abdominal pain
A proportion of patients admit to a stressful event associated with the onset of pain and/or exacerbating existing pain. Many patients complain of pain after a meal and

this may be due to the gastrocolic reflex. In patients with IBS the gastrocolic reflex is more pronounced, delayed and often associated with pain. Night pain is not a feature of IBS, although pain on awakening is well documented. The location of the abdominal pain is not specific and may occur in any area of the abdomen, although the common site is the left lower quadrant of the abdomen. The severity of pain may range from cutting, cramping pain that doubles the patient up, to a background ache not interfering with daily activities. During a single episode, the pain could fluctuate. The duration of pain is variable from short episodes to continuous pain lasting days or even weeks.

Factors that relieve the pain are inconsistent and include a bowel action or the passage of wind from either mouth or anus. It is frequently observed that abdominal pain is associated with abdominal distension. Patients with severe pain may require potent analgesics for relief.

The mechanism of pain is not well understood despite numerous studies. Studies on motor activity are contradictory: both increased and decreased activity are documented. It is also suggested that pain occurring after food is mediated by hormones. Gastrin and cholecystokinin are both released postprandially and stimulate the intestine muscle.

Altered bowel habits

An altered bowel habit is a prerequisite symptom for the diagnosis of IBS. Patients with IBS have bowel dysfunction similar to the normal population but the response is disproportionate. Disordered bowel habit consists of diarrhoea and constipation. There are more complaints of constipation in the elderly.

Diarrhoea is commonly characterized by small volume, frequent motions. Although the definition of diarrhoea, as three or more loose bowel actions per day, is fulfilled it is interesting that in many studies the 24 h stool weight is normal.

The stools of patients with IBS who are constipated are described as 'rabbit droppings', 'goat droppings', ribbon-like, hard balls or pellets. Frequent questioning on the nature of a patient's stools may cause anxiety when the perceived ideal stool is not seen.

Abdominal distension

The cause of abdominal distension in IBS is not documented. The report that patients with IBS do not have increased gas in the gastrointestinal tract is unconfirmed. Gas in the alimentary tract derives from two sources: swallowed air and endogenous production. Excessive air swallowing is usually due to anxiety. Contributory factors to air swallowing include: ill-fitting dentures, chewing gum, irritative mouth lesions, orthodontic appliances and hypersalivation: 2–3 ml of air enters the stomach at each swallow and more air is swallowed with liquids and solids. Aerophagy is increased with dysphagia or odynophagia. Lactose intolerance, malabsorption syndromes and bacterial overgrowth of the small intestine are associated with flatulence.

Other symptoms

Studies have established that IBS patients are more likely than controls to suffer from back pain, headache, tiredness, an unpleasant taste in the mouth, dyspareunia, urinary frequency, urgency, nocturia and incomplete emptying of the bladder.

Physical examination

Physical examination is unrevealing apart from the frequent, though not inevitable, finding of abdominal tenderness over the colon. In some patients the entire palpable length of the colon is tender. The sigmoid and descending colon are usually the most tender areas. Patients may complain that the pain during deep palpation is similar to what they experience during an attack.

A rectal examination and sigmoidoscopy are important. Sigmoidoscopy is valuable both diagnostically and therapeutically. Information that there is no malignancy is reassuring to the patient.

Diagnosis

In medical practice most diseases are diagnosed on symptoms and aetiology, supported by evidence from investigations. In IBS the diagnosis is based on at least a three-month history of abdominal pain and/or altered bowel habit and abdominal distension.

Diagnostic criteria of IBS

Abdominal pain relieved by defaecation and/or altered defaecation (with two or more of the following):

- altered stool frequency
- altered stool form
- altered stool passage (straining or urgency; feeling of incomplete evacuation)
- passage of mucus associated usually with abdominal distension.

These diagnostic criteria correlate with the findings of Manning and colleagues (1978) who established that: 'Four symptoms were significantly more common among patients with IBS – namely distension, relief of pain with bowel movement, and looser and more frequent bowel movements with the onset of pain. Mucus and a sensation of incomplete evacuation were also common in these patients.' Radiological, endoscopic and laboratory investigations are normal.

Any elderly patient who complains of abdominal pain, flatulence and a persistent erratic bowel pattern should have a detailed medical and psychosocial evaluation, including investigations, laboratory tests and specialist consultation. A guideline for diagnostic evaluation is:

- history
- physical examination
- pelvic examination
- sigmoidoscopy
- stool testing
- full blood count
- urinalysis
- thyroid function tests.

Some advocate the diagnosis of IBS on the basis of exclusion of other disease entities with a similar clinical profile. Others advocate a positive diagnosis on the basis of a careful history, physical examination and investigations. Retrospective evaluation of patients who were diagnosed as IBS, suffering from abdominal pain and diarrhoea, included many with lactose intolerance, and this condition may need to be excluded. At present no diagnostic test is available to make a diagnosis of IBS.

Management

Elderly patients with IBS are likely to have seen many medical practitioners with little or no relief of their symptoms and possibly told that 'nothing is wrong', 'nothing abnormal was found', 'it's your nerves' or 'the pain is in your mind'. Frequently, elderly IBS patients are frustrated, resigned or demoralized. They may have experienced overt or covert rejection and view doctors as uncaring or incompetent. Some elderly IBS patients may harbour the fear that the doctors may have missed a malignancy, especially if history taking and physical examination were hurried.

It is essential at initial contact to establish a positive working relationship with the patient. A comprehensive, detailed history and physical examination will communicate interest and reassure the patient that nothing significant is missed.

A comprehensive detailed history will also reveal the treatments which have been used previously and the patient's compliance with treatment.

Time spent with a patient also conveys the physician's acceptance of the illness and will allay the patient's fear of rejection. When feelings of acceptance and support are established, the patient's frustration and demoralization will diminish. In addition, a detailed history inspires confidence in the physician. This will lay the ground work for the patient to later accept the doctor's diagnosis of IBS.

Some IBS patients do not report events which others would experience as psychologically stressful. They do not consciously feel emotionally perturbed by these events. On the other hand, when they experience stress, they are unable to express these events as emotionally distressing. These patients are called alexithymic and have difficulty in identifying psychosocial stressors in their lives. The physician should persist in attempting to identify psychosocial stressors which are not readily disclosed. Some IBS patients may have a tendency to present an unrealistically positive, well adjusted manner; others with major depressive disorders do not view themselves as depressed.

Referral to a psychiatrist is necessary if there is a definite link between psychosocial stressors and onset or exacerbation of IBS symptoms, or if there is a psychiatric disorder present concurrently with IBS symptoms. This is often a difficult task to accomplish as the patient must not be made to feel abandoned. It is important for the physician to discuss the reasons for the referral in terms of benefit to the patient. This should be done by showing compassion for the patient's suffering, stressing that the symptoms are real and that psychological factors may contribute to the symptoms. Feelings of rejection or abandonment can be allayed and continuing interest emphasized by making a firm appointment to review the patient after the visit to the psychiatrist.

The patient with IBS has other hurdles to clear. A major one is what to convey to members of the family, friends and colleagues. What did the doctor find? What did the tests show?

It is not easy for patients (or for doctors for that matter) to understand IBS. It is even more difficult for the patient to explain IBS to others, particularly to those sceptical that nothing was ever wrong! The patient must be given a clear, simple 'take home message'. The simple diagram of the colon drawn in a normal state and in spasm is useful, with the analogy that the pain in the colon is similar to a 'cramp' in the calf muscle.

The patient's understanding that there is no 'quick cure' is essential. Unrealistic expectations can lead to hostility towards the doctor. Since the IBS is notoriously difficult to cure this must be emphasized.

In an authoritative review of drug therapy in IBS, Klein (1988) reported placebo responses in excess of 70 per cent and concluded: 'In my opinion not a single study has been published that provides compelling evidence that any therapeutic agent is efficacious in the global treatment of IBS. This is not to say that no effective therapies exist; only that none have been documented'. High fibre diets were prescribed in the treatment of IBS and initial enthusiasm has waned in the wake of controlled trials. This type of diet may have some placebo value and helps with constipation. It is important to note that excess fibre can increase the frequency of bowel actions and flatulence.

It is important that spurious diarrhoea due to constipation be diagnosed and treated. Therapy should be directed towards pain relief (antispasmodic drugs) and diarrhoea (loperamide, diphenoxylate). Peppermint oil has no proven benefit. Some patients are helped by a combination of mebeverine hydrochloride and an antidepressant.

Psychosocial treatment appears to have variable success rates. In most cases it would be difficult to explain to the patient that he needed or could benefit from psychological or behavioural management. In those patients where psychosocial stressors are clearly delineated to be associated with exacerbation of their symptoms, various psychosocial treatments can be beneficial. These include relaxation techniques and stress management, biofeedback training, cognitive behaviour therapy, supportive psychotherapy, hypnotherapy and psychodynamic psychotherapy.

Hypnotherapy and psychodynamic psychotherapy have been used successfully in treating patients with chronic refractory IBS and may be considered as an adjunct to medical management.

A detailed history from IBS patients may often reveal the occurrence of psychosocial stressors associated with the onset of symptoms. The symptoms experienced by the elderly patients with IBS are similar to those of younger patients with the triad of abdominal pain, altered bowel habit and abdominal distension being most prominent.

The physician can confidently make a diagnosis from the history, physical examination and a few simple diagnostic investigations. Management is directed primarily towards relief of symptoms, identifying factors which possibly aggravate the disorder and helping the patient adjust to what is often a chronic relapsing condition.

BIBLIOGRAPHY AND FURTHER READING

Chaudhary, N.A. & Truelove, S.C. (1962). The irritable colon syndrome: a study of the clinical features, predisposing causes and prognosis in 130 cases. *Q. J. Med.* **31**:307–22.

Craig, T.K. & Brown, G.W. (1984). Goal frustration and life events in the aetiology of painful gastrointestinal disorder. *J. Psychosom. Res.* **28**:411–21.

Esler, M.D. & Goulston, K.J. (1973). Levels of anxiety and colonic disorders. *N. Engl. J. Med.* **288**:16–20.

Ford, M.J., Millar, P.M., Eastwood, J. & Eastwood, M.A. (1987). Life events, psychiatric illness and the irritable bowel syndrome. *Gut* **28**:160–5.

Greenbaum, D.S. (1984). Preliminary report on anti-depressant treatment of irritable bowel syndrome: comments on comparison with anxiolytic therapy. *Psychopharmacol. Bull.* **20**:622–8.

Grundy, D. (1991). Involvement of extrinsic nerves in functional disorders of the bowel. In *Irritable Bowel Syndrome*, ed. N.W. Read, pp. 51–7. London: Blackwell.

Heaton, K.W. (1988). Functional bowel disease. In *Recent Advances in Gastroenterology*, ed. R.E. Pounder, pp. 291–312. Edinburgh: Churchill Livingstone.

Hislop, I.G. (1971). Psychological significance of the irritable colon syndrome. *Gut* 12:452–7.

Kellow, J.E. & Evans, P.R. (1993). Management of irritable bowel syndrome. *J. Gastroenterol. Hepatol.* 8:287–93.

Klein, K.B. (1988). Controlled treatment trials in the irritable bowel syndrome: a critique. *Gastroenterology* 95:232–41.

Lynn, R.B. & Friedman, L.S. (1993). Irritable bowel syndrome. *N. Engl. J. Med.* 329:1940–5.

Manning, A.P., Thompson, W.G., Heaton, K.W. & Morris, A.F. (1978). Towards positive diagnosis of the irritable bowel. *Br. Med. J.* 2:653–4.

O'Keefe, E. & Talley, N.J. (1991). Irritable bowel syndrome in the elderly. *Clin. Geriatr. Med.* 7:265–86.

Talley, N.J., O'Keefe, E.A., Zinsmeister, A.R. & Melton, L.J. III (1992). Prevalence of gastrointestinal symptoms in the elderly: a population-based study. *Gastroenterology* 102:895–901.

Toner, B.B., Garfinkel, P.E., Jeejeebhoy, K.N., Scher, H., Shulhan D. & Di-Gasbarro I. (1990). Self-schemia in irritable bowel syndrome. *Psychosom. Med.* 52:149–55.

Wender, P.H. & Kalm, M. (1983). Prevalence of attention deficit disorder, residual type, and other psychiatric disorders in patients with irritable bowel syndrome. *Am. J. Psychiatry* 140:1579–82.

Whitcomb, F.F. & Cain, J.C. (1963). Irritable bowel. *Postgrad. Med.* 33:233–6.

Whorwell, P.J. (1991). Extraintestinal manifestations of the irritable bowel syndrome. In *Irritable Bowel Syndrome*, ed. N.W. Read, pp. 43–7. London: Blackwell.

Ranjit N. Ratnaike, Joseph E. Buttery and David J. Torpy

Diarrhoea may be a consequence of endocrine disorders, hormone-secreting tumours, metabolic illnesses and a variety of miscellaneous conditions.

Hyperthyroidism

Between 15 and 18 per cent of patients with thyrotoxicosis are above the age of 60 years. There is a female predominance of four to one.

Only about 25 per cent of elderly patients with thyrotoxicosis manifest the disease clinically. In the majority the presentation is that of 'apathetic hyperthyroidism' a term coined by Lahey in 1931, and characterized by lethargy and apathy, and the absence of eye signs and tachycardia. Cardiovascular effects such as atrial fibrillation and the attendent risk of embolism produce the most frequent and severe morbidity in this age group. Occasionally, diarrhoea attributed to gastrointestinal hypermotility may be the only symptom and of sufficient severity to cause dehydration and hypokalaemia. In a number of patients steatorrhoea is present. The mechanism is unknown.

Hypothyroidism

In the elderly patient the symptoms of hypothyroidism are insidious and may be present for years before the diagnosis is made. Constipation is the pre-eminent gastrointestinal symptom. Diarrhoea sometimes occurs and may be associated with malabsorption and steatorrhoea. Decreased intestinal motility and prolonged intestinal transit time could predispose to small intestinal bacterial overgrowth and diarrhoea (see Chapter 9).

Diabetes mellitus

Diabetes mellitus is common in the elderly. Diarrhoea in patients with diabetes mellitus is well documented, especially in those on insulin treatment with poorly controlled blood glucose or evidence of peripheral vascular disease and neuropathy. Diabetic diarrhoea is classically nocturnal, though not invariably so.

Diarrhoea is attributed to an autonomic neuropathy causing both decreased and increased motility. Although abnormalities in motility are not in dispute the mechanism of diarrhoea is uncertain. It is suggested that, in patients with slow intestinal transit, diarrhoea is due to bacterial overgrowth. In others, diarrhoea is a result of 'rapid' transit.

The autonomic nervous system is also associated with intestinal absorption and secretion. The role of α_2 adrenergic receptors in the intestinal transport of ions is well established. These receptors are present on the enterocytes, and stimulation leads to increased fluid and electrolyte absorption and the inhibition of secretion. In diabetics with severe autonomic neuropathy, diarrhoea is due to net fluid secretion. Treatment with α_2 adrenergic agonists such as clonidine and lidamidine is beneficial. These agents decrease cyclic AMP concentrations in the enterocyte, and net water and electrolyte retention occurs. Unfortunately, central nervous and cardiovascular system side-effects, particularly in the elderly, limit their usefulness.

It would seem that the mechanism of diarrhoea in patients with diabetes mellitus is multifactorial. Although conclusive data is lacking, the rigorous control of blood glucose levels may have a beneficial effect on the control of diarrhoea. The presence of an associated upper gastrointestinal motility disorder may make good glycaemic control more difficult.

Pancreatic disease

In the elderly, despite the decline in pancreatic secretory function with age, steatorrhoea is not a consequence, as loss of 90 per cent pancreatic secretory function is necessary for steatorrhoea to occur. However, pancreatic insufficiency is the most common cause of steatorrhoea in the elderly. Steatorrhoea is a frequent feature of chronic pancreatitis but not of pancreatic carcinoma. Alcoholic and idiopathic pancreatitis comprise about 95 per cent of cases of chronic pancreatitis. In the elderly a common form of pancreatitis is a subtype of nonalcoholic pancreatitis termed 'idiopathic senile chronic pancreatitis'. In one large series the incidence of steatorrhoea was 71 per cent, and occurred well before the onset of diabetes mellitus. Epigastric pain and pancreatic calcification were not prominent features. There is evidence that the risk factors associated with arteriosclerosis are common to idiopathic senile chronic pancreatitis.

The characteristic feature of chronic pancreatitis is recurrent attacks of severe pain, located in the epigastrium and frequently referred to the back. The intensity of the pain varies with posture and is relieved by bending forward. A diagnosis of chronic pancreatitis should be considered in patients with a history of recurrent upper abdominal pain with diarrhoea associated with steatorrhoea, weight loss and diabetes mellitus. In this clinical setting, pancreatic calcification and a normal small bowel biopsy strongly suggest a pancreatic cause of diarrhoea.

Carcinoma of the pancreas

In the differential diagnosis of steatorrhoea due to a pancreatic cause, the condition of chronic primary inflammatory pancreatitis should be considered. This entity, although very uncommon, occurs in elderly females and the clinical features are diarrhoea, weight loss, mild abdominal pain and, occasionally, pyrexia. There is neither diabetes mellitus nor pancreatic calcification.

The incidence of carcinoma of the pancreas is increasing and it is the fourth most common cause of death due a malignancy in the UK and USA. At diagnosis most patients are over the age of 60 years, with a male predominance.

The clinical features vary with the site of the carcinoma. In carcinoma of the head of the pancreas and ampulla of Vater, the prominent feature is jaundice. Carcinoma of the body or tail of the pancreas manifests upper abdominal pain that 'bores' to the back, changes with position and is relieved on leaning forward. Diabetes mellitus is a frequent complication.

Prompt investigation with CT scanning is warranted since early surgical resection is curative. Unfortunately, few patients have resectable lesions at the time of diagnosis. In inoperable cases, combined chemotherapy and radiotherapy are palliative.

Gastrinoma

Gastrinomas are nonbeta cell islet cell tumours that secrete gastrin, found mostly in the duodenal wall or pancreas. The Zollinger–Ellison syndrome consists of a nonbeta islet cell tumour of the pancreas, hypersecretion of gastric acid and peptic ulcer disease. Z–E syndrome can occur as an isolated phenomenon or as part of the multiple endocrine neoplasia type I (MEN-I) syndrome, an autosomal dominant disorder characterized by endocrine tumours of the pituitary gland, pancreas and parathyroids, as well as other manifestations including lipomata and, less commonly, tumours of other organs such as the adrenals and thyroid gland. MEN-I is due to a mutation of the recently isolated MENIN gene located on chromosome 11 (11q13).

Diarrhoea may be the initial feature. The steatorrhoea which often accompanies the diarrhoea is secondary to pancreatic lipase inactivation and bile salt precipitation in the duodenum as a result of the large load of gastric acid which enters the intestine. Villous atrophy of the small intestinal mucosa, due to the excessive acid secretion, contributes to the steatorrhoea.

Gastrinoma is confirmed by a raised plasma gastrin concentration with high acid secretion. Intravenous administration of secretin causes a substantial increase in serum gastrin concentrations. The tumours occur within the duodenal wall, the pancreas or may be found elsewhere in metastatic cases. Multiple tumours are common particularly in MEN-I cases. Octreotide scintigraphy, which labels somatostatin receptors in vivo, is the most sensitive noninvasive tumour localization technique. Anatomical definition can be obtained with CT or MRI scanning.

Acid reduction is now achieved with omeprazole. The drug is safe and well tolerated, and is the treatment of choice for increased acid secretion in gastrinoma. Treatment of hypercalcaemia, from hyperparathyroidism, in MEN-I cases may help control acid hypersecretion. Larger tumours should be considered for excision on the basis of malignant potential. Treatment with octreotide and chemotherapy with streptozocin, 5-fluorouracil and doxorubicin have been advocated for metastatic gastrinoma with some success. Since gastric acid secretion can now be readily controlled with proton pump inhibitors such as omeprazole, the prognosis depends largely on the metastatic potential of the gastrinoma tumours.

Carcinoid tumours

Carcinoid tumours are uncommon, comprising about 0.5–1 per cent of gastrointestinal tumours. They may originate from the foregut, midgut or hindgut. Carcinoid tumours can occur at any age, the peak incidence being between 50 and 60 years for all tumour sites except the appendix.

The tumours produce serotonin (5-hydroxytryptamine) and other peptide mediators such as somatostatin, kinins, prostaglandins, adrenocorticotropin, histamine and substance P.

Only about 5 per cent of patients with carcinoid tumours show any symptoms. Serotonin overproduction is characterized by flushing, diarrhoea, cardiac fibrosis and pellagra dermatosis (due to niacin deficiency). Diarrhoea is the second most prominent symptom after flushing in the carcinoid syndrome. The diarrhoea is explosive and watery. Serotonin increases the intracytosolic Ca in the enterocyte which then leads to a secretory diarrhoea.

The diagnosis is made by an elevated 24 h urine 5-hydroxyindoleacetic acid (5-HIAA), the major metabolite of serotonin. The flush provocative test with an intravenous injection of epinephrine has been used but is of limited value because of potential hazard to the patient and equivocal results.

The treatment of choice is surgical resection if the tumour is in the foregut. Tumours in other sites are associated with hepatic metastases and treatment consists of percutaneous hepatic arterial devascularization and chemotherapy.

The synthetic antioestrogen drug, tamoxifen, is reported to cause improvement in 5-HIAA excretion and tumour regression in one study, but was ineffectual in another study.

Octreotide, a somatostatin analogue, is effective in controlling flushing and diarrhoea. There is also a decrease in the 5-HIAA excretion and, in some instances, tumour mass reduction.

Medullary thyroid carcinoma

Medullary thyroid carcinoma (MTC) comprises approximately 5 to 10 per cent of all thyroid malignancies. MTC may occur sporadically or as a component of the multiple endocrine neoplasia type IIa (MEN-II) syndrome, comprising MTC, primary hyperparathyroidism and phaeochromocytoma. Patients with the MEN-IIb syndrome also develop MTC but not hyperparathyroidism, and have characteristic mucosal neuromas of the lips and, sometimes, a marfanoid appearance. MTC may also be familial without the other features of MEN-II. All these familial syndromes are autosomal dominant and due to different mutations of the RET-proto-oncogene. RET mutation testing allows prevention of MTC by thyroidectomy of young children in affected families. MTC can occur in the young and in the elderly with no predilection for either sex. There are no reliable data on the incidence of MTC in the elderly. The humoral messengers produced by MTC, calcitonin, serotonin, prostaglandins, somatostatin, calcitonin, kallikrein, motilin, substance P and bombesin may be involved in the pathogenesis of diarrhoea which is secretory in nature.

The most common symptom is diarrhoea in 30 to 40 per cent of patients with MTC and is related to the size of the tumour mass. The most common presentation is a thyroid nodule. The tumour usually runs a slow but progressive course. The neck structures are invaded and metastases to the cervical lymph nodules and distant sites, such as the lung, liver, bone and adrenal glands, can occur.

An increase in plasma calcitonin concentration after the intravenous infusion of calcium or pentagastrin, or both, have been used to predict MTC in familial cases although mutation screening is more reliable and offers earlier diagnosis.

The treatment is surgical in the early stages of MTC when the neoplasm is confined to the thyroid gland. In patients with inoperable or recurrent disease, no particular therapy is proven effective. The tumour does not concentrate radioactive iodine.

Antimotility drugs such as loperamide are useful in the management of mild diarrhoea. Although the diarrhoea is secretory, octreotide is not reliably effective.

Somatostatinoma

The peak incidence is in the fifth decade and males and females are affected equally. This extremely rare tumuor contains or secretes excessive amounts of somatostatin, a 14 or 28 amino acid peptide.

Patients with somatostatinomas present with diabetes mellitus, gallbladder disease, diarrhoea, weight loss and anaemia. Pancreatic somatostatinomas, however, are associated with a higher prevalence of diarrhoea than the intestinal variety. The diarrhoea is thought to be secondary to the pancreatic insufficiency and decreased bile acid output. Consequently, steatorrhoea often accompanies the diarrhoea.

The diagnosis is based on an elevated plasma somatostatin concentration, usually in patients with large pancreatic tumours and those with metastases in the liver, but not in patients with small duodenal somatostatinomas. Most pancreatic primary tumours are large and can be detected by CT scan, angiography or ultrasound.

Treatment is by surgical removal of the tumour where feasible and, in approximately 50 per cent of cases, this may result in a cure. Chemotherapy may be of benefit in selected patients with liver metastases.

Glucagonoma

This is a rare tumour of the alpha cells of the islets of Langerhans which secrete glucagon. Most cases occur in the middle aged or elderly and the average age of onset is about 55 years. Both sexes are equally affected.

The most common site for the tumour is at the tail of the pancreas but may arise from any location in the pancreas. Glucagon, a polypeptide of 29 amino acids, acts to increase blood glucose concentration.

The most characteristic feature of glucagonoma is the presence of necrolytic migratory erythematous rash. Patients are usually mildly diabetic with little or no diabetic complications or ketoacidosis. Weight loss and diarrhoea are also seen. The diarrhoea may cause hypokalaemia. Steatorrhoea is usually minimal or absent.

Diagnosis is based on an elevated fasting plasma glucagon concentration, which may be 10 to 20 times normal. The tumour can be localized with CT scanning, but selective angiography is often used to augment CT scanning.

Surgical excision of the tumour, even when metastases are present, improves the condition of the patient. Chemotherapy has limited success.

VIPoma

The VIPoma is a tumour in the pancreas which produces excessive vasoactive intestinal peptide (VIP). About half of all VIPomas are benign. The features of excessive VIP production are watery diarrhoea, hypokalaemia and achlorhydria (the WDHA syndrome; Verner–Morrison syndrome; pancreatic cholera). Most patients with VIPoma are hypochlorhydric and not achlorhydric. The profuse diarrhoea can result in dehydration, hypokalaemia and metabolic acidosis. In the elderly, in addition to diarrhoea, faecal incontinence occurs due to the direct action of VIP on internal sphincter pressure.

An elevated plasma VIP concentration is diagnostic of VIPoma. The pancreatic tumour can be identified by selective angiography, abdominal ultrasonography and CT scanning.

The replacement of fluid and electrolyte losses, especially potassium, is important in the immediate treatment of severe diarrhoea to prevent complications from hypovolaemia and hypokalaemia. Intravenous fluids in excess of 6 l/day and potassium supplements of about 35 mmol/day may be necessary. Surgical removal of the tumour is the most definitive treatment, but may not be feasible. With diffuse islet cell hyperplasia, partial or complete pancreatectomy may be carried out. Patients with inoperable tumours can have debulking operations or chemotherapy. The response to chemotherapy using the combination of 5-fluorouracil and streptozocin is effective in lowering VIP levels and lessening the diarrhoea.

The most potent natural antagonist of VIPomas is somatostatin, but its clinical usefulness is limited because of its short half-life of 1.5 min. which necessitates intravenous administration. The somatostatin analogue, octreotide, is now the drug of choice in the management of VIP-associated diarrhoea. In addition, this drug is said to reduce tumour size in some patients.

Systemic mastocytosis

Systemic mastocytosis is the abnormal accumulation of mast cells in the liver, spleen, bone marrow, bone and gastrointestinal tract. Infiltration of mast cells into specific organs causes organomegaly. About 25 to 50 per cent of patients with systemic mastocytosis suffer from gastrointestinal symptoms which include vomiting, diarrhoea and malabsorption, and abdominal pain. The diarrhoea can be intermittent or more permanent and associated with steatorrhoea. Attacks of flushing occur.

The diagnosis is based on the histological confirmation of increased numbers of mast cells in a small bowel biopsy with mild villous atrophy. Suspected proliferation of mast cells in bone can be identified from radionuclide bone scan.

The diarrhoea is controlled by the administration of an H_2 histamine receptor antagonist and disodium cromoglycate.

Iatrogenic causes of diarrhoea

Gastrointestinal surgery

Diarrhoea complicates a variety of gastrointestinal surgical procedures. Surgery to decrease gastric acid production, performed in the past on patients with peptic ulcer disease, may cause diarrhoea. Mild postvagotomy diarrhoea occurs in about 70 per cent of subjects and severe diarrhoea in 5 to 20 per cent. The mechanism of diarrhoea is speculative. The most probable explanation is that diarrhoea is secondary to deconjugation of bile salts due to bacterial overgrowth from decreased gastric acidity. Other contributory factors to diarrhoea are rapid gastric emptying, accelerated transit of intestinal contents or an increased fluid volume to the colon. Diarrhoea after a partial gastrectomy is due to increased transit time and this has been documented by the hydrogen breath test. The view that diarrhoea is more frequently associated with postvagotomy in comparison with partial gastrectomy is no longer sustained on the basis of recent research.

Diarrhoea also occurs after colonic resection, depending on the length of colon removed, due to a reduction in colonic absorptive capacity and possible derangement of colonic motility. Ileal resection of less than 100 cm may be associated with diarrhoea. Decreased absorption of bile acids imposes a greater load on the colon where, notably, dihydroxy bile acids induce increased fluid and electrolyte secretion. In patients with a resection of more than 100 cm of the ileum, the enterohepatic circulation which reabsorbs about 90 per cent of bile acids is deranged and the bile acid pool is severely depleted. Consequently, fat malabsorption and steatorrhoea result.

The role of the ileocaecal valve in maintaining the sterility of the small bowel is now under question. The absence of the ileocaecal valve, no longer acting as a 'brake' to the entry of ileal contents to the colon, may result in some degree of diarrhoea.

Postcholecystectomy diarrhoea is well documented and has traditionally been attributed to the effects of bile acids. However, in the majority of postcholecystectomy patients a link between the secretory effects of bile acids and diarrhoea has not been established.

Radiation enteritis

Diarrhoea is a common side-effect of radiation therapy for malignancies in the elderly such as carcinoma of the cervix, uterus, rectum and prostate. The availability of supravoltage radiation which delivers high doses of radiation with minimal or absent skin has increased gastrointestinal problems such as diarrhoea. The small intestine is particularly vulnerable to ionizing radiation due to the rapid turnover of the epithelial cells. Damage to the less mobile duodenum and terminal ileum results in bacterial overgrowth diarrhoea, malabsorption and stricture formation. In the colon, as the caecum and rectosigmoid are fixed in the pelvis they experience more mucosal damage which may cause bleeding. About 50 per cent of patients may experience diarrhoea. In both the small and large intestine diarrhoea may occur soon after therapy, often with spontaneous recovery. In about 10 per cent of patients, diarrhoea may occur even after two to three decades due to chronic radiation damage.

Intestinal pseudo-obstruction

Intestinal pseudo-obstruction is a condition of chronic bowel obstruction in the absence of a demonstrable mechanical cause. Primary intestinal pseudo-obstruction is due to degenerative changes in the myenteric plexus of the intestine and this results in a dysfunction in intestinal motility.

Vomiting, abdominal pain and, in a subset of patients, dysphagia are significant problems. Due to the motor disorder of the intestine, bacterial overgrowth and its consequences, diarrhoea and steatorrhoea, and vitamin B_{12} and folate deficiencies are possible complications. Barium studies demonstrate distension of segments of the small intestine or colon.

Secondary intestinal pseudo-obstruction occurs due to systemic and local diseases and drug therapy.

Systemic diseases
- Diabetes mellitus
- Hypothyroidism
- Amyloidosis
- Scleroderma
- Polymyositis
- Parkinson's disease.

Local causes
- Coeliac disease
- Chagas' disease
- Cathartic colon.

Therapeutic agents
- Tricyclic antidepressants
- Phenothiazines.

Lactose intolerance

The most common cause of carbohydrate malabsorption is lactose intolerance due to an absence or deficiency of the enzyme lactase in the small intestine.

In lactose intolerance the disaccharidase lactase, a brush border enzyme, acts on lactose:

$$\text{Lactose} \xrightarrow{\text{lactase}} \text{glucose} + \text{galactose}$$

If lactase is absent or depleted, the undigested lactose reaches the colon unchanged and is metabolized by colonic bacteria:

$$\text{Lactose} \xrightarrow{\text{colonic bacteria}} \text{acetic, propionic and butyric acids}$$

These organic acids, acetate, propionate and butyrate, act as osmotic agents.

The clinical diagnosis is based on explosive watery diarrhoea, cramping abdominal pain, abdominal distension and flatulence after the ingestion of milk or milk products. Interestingly, yoghurt may be consumed with no ill effects since bacterial lactase in yoghurt is activated at body temperature.

Lactase deficiency is primary or secondary. The incidence of lactase deficiency in the elderly is not known. It is likely that secondary lactose intolerance, rather than the congenital primary form, is more common. Secondary lactose intolerance, which is mild and temporary, occurs frequently as a result of damage to the small intestinal villi due to infection, radiation therapy or a primary mucosal disorder such as coeliac disease.

After a bacterial infection of the small intestine, or when coeliac disease is diagnosed and a gluten-free diet introduced, milk and milk products should be avoided for a short period (e.g. one week) until the concentration of lactase reverts to normal. In the enterocyte, maximum lactase concentrations are reached when the enterocytes which clothe the villi reach a mid-villus position during their movement from the crypt to the tip of the villus where they are extruded.

Although the diagnosis of lactose intolerance is possible in children, on the basis of reducing substances present in the stools (before or after acid hydrolysis) and decreasing the faecal pH, in adults with lactose intolerance the stool pH is normal. The diagnosis is made by the hydrogen breath test in preference to an oral lactose tolerance test or the quantification of lactase in a specimen of small bowel mucosa.

A cheap, rapid visual screening test is now available.

Eosinophilic gastroenteritis

This is an uncommon entity due to diffuse infiltration of eosinophils in the gastric antrum, small intestine and colon. The aetiology is unclear. In patients with predominantly small intestinal involvement, the presenting symptoms are abdominal pain, diarrhoea associated with steatorrhoea, and a protein-losing enteropathy. The distinctive small bowel feature is clumps of eosinophils within the lamina propria; villous atrophy can be severe. Blood eosinophilia is a constant feature. Steroids are helpful in the management and if obstructive symptoms occur surgical intervention is required.

BIBLIOGRAPHY AND FURTHER READING

Carcinoid tumours

Boden, G. & Shelmet, J.J. (1987). Gastrointestinal hormones and the carcinoid tumors and syndrome. In *Endocrinology and Metabolism*, 2nd edn, ed. P. Felig, J.D. Baxter, A.E. Broadus & L.A. Frohman, pp. 1629–62. New York: McGraw-Hill.

Kvols, L.K. (1989). Therapy of the malignant carcinoid syndrome. *Endocrinol. Metab. Clin. North Am.* **18**:557–68.

Maton, P.N. (1990). The carcinoid tumor and the carcinoid syndrome. In *Principles and Practice of Endocrinology and Metabolism*, ed. K.L. Becker, pp 1640–3. Philadelphia: Lippincott.

Vinik, A.I., McLeod, M.K., Fig, L.M., Shapiro, B., Lloyd, R.V. & Cho, K. (1989) Clinical features, diagnosis and localization of carcinoid tumors and their management. *Gastroenterol. Clin. North Am.* **18**:865–96.

Diabetes mellitus

Beebe, D.K. & Walley, E. (1992). Diabetic diarrhoea: an underdiagnosed complication? *Postgrad. Med.* **91**:179–86.

Chang, E.B., Bergenstal, R.M. & Field, M. (1985). Diarrhoea in streptozocin-treated rats. Loss of adrenergic regulation of intestinal fluid and electrolyte transport. *J. Clin. Invest.* **75**:1666–70.

Chang, E.B. & Fedorak, R.N. (1991). Diabetic diarrhoea. In *Diarrhoeal Diseases*, ed. M. Field, pp. 413–27. New York: Elsevier.

Schiller, L.R. & Feldman, M. (1990). Gastrointestinal complications of diabetes. In *Principles and Practice of Endocrinology and Metabolism*, ed. K.L. Becker, pp 1144–7. Philadelphia: Lippincott.

Eosinophilic gastroenteritis

Sawaya, S.M., Misk, R.J. & Aftimos, G.P. (1992). Eosinophilic gastroenteritis: report of two cases and comment on the literature. *Eur. J. Surg.* **158**:439–41.

Gastrinoma

Berg, C.L. & Wolfe, M.M. (1991). Zollinger-Ellison syndrome. *Med. Clin. North Am.* **75**:903–21.

Bloom, S.R. & Polak, J.M. (1990). The endocrine gastrointestinal tract: tumors. In *Principles and Practice of Endocrinology and Metabolism*, ed. K.L. Becker, pp 1337–42. Philadelphia: Lippincott.

Chandrasekharappa, S.C., Guru, S.C., Manickam, P. et al. (1997). Positional cloning of the gene for multiple endocrine neoplasia type 1. *Science* **276** (5311):404–7.

Jensen, R.T. & Fraker D.L. (1994). Zollinger–Ellison syndrome. Advances in treatment of gastric hypersecretion and the gastrinoma. *J. Am. Med. Assoc.* **271**:1429–35.

Vinayek, R., Frucht, H., Chiang, H.C., Maton, P.N., Gardner, J.D. & Jensen, R.T. (1990). Zollinger–Ellison syndrome: Recent advances in the management of gastrinoma. *Gastrenterol. Clin. North Am.* **19**:197–217.

Gastrointestinal surgery

Beckwith, P.S., Wolff, B.G. & Frazee, R.C. (1992). Ileorectostomy in the older patient. *Dis. Colon Rectum* **35**:301–4.

Bond, J.H. & Levitt, M.D. (1977). Use of breath hydrogen [H2] to quantitate small bowel transit time following partial gastrectomy. *J. Lab. Clin. Med.* **90**:30–6.

Cox, A.G. (1970). Vagotomy and drainage procedures: the present position. *Prog. Surg.* **8**:45–68.

Fromm, H., Tunuguntla, A.K., Malavolti, M., Sherman, C. & Ceryak, S. (1987). Absence of significant role of bile salts in diarrhoea of a heterogeneous group of postcholecystectomy patients. *Dig. Dis. Sci.* **32**:33–44.

Jordan, P.H. & Condon, R.E. (1970). A prospective evaluation of vagotomy-pyloroplasty and vagotomy-antrectomy for treatment of duodenal ulcer. *Ann. Surg.* **172**:547–63

Glucagonoma

Bloom, S.R. & Polak, J.M. (1990). The endocrine gastrointestinal tract: tumors. In *Principles and Practice of Endocrinology and Metabolism*, ed. K.L. Becker, pp 1337–42. Philadelphia: Lippincott.

Vinik, A.I. & Moattari, A.R. (1989). Treatment of endocrine tumors of the pancreas. *Endocrinol. Metab. Clin. North Am.* **18**:483–518.

Hyperthyroidism

Bayer, M.F. (1991). Effective laboratory evaluation of thyroid status. *Med. Clin. North Am.* **75**:1–26.

Burman, K.D. (1990). Hyperthyroidism. In *Principles and Practice of Endocrinology and Metabolism*, ed. K.L. Becker, pp 331–47. Philadelphia: Lippincott.

Intestinal pseudo-obstruction

Dawson, D.J., Sciberras, C.M. & Whitwell, H. (1984). Coeliac disease presenting with intestinal pseudo-obstruction. *Gut* **25**:1003–8.

Lactose intolerance

Caspary, W.F. (1986). Diarrhoea associated with carbohydrate malabsorption. *Clin. Gastroenterol.* **15**:631–55.

Buttery, J.E., Ratnaike, R.N. & Chamberlain, B.R. (1994). A visual screening method for lactose maldigestion. *Ann. Clin. Biochem.* **31**:566–7.

Kolars, J.C., Levitt, M.D., Aouji, M. & Savaiano, D.A. (1984). Yoghurt – an autodigesting source of lactose. *N. Engl. J. Med.* **310**:1–3.

Medullary thyroid carcinoma

Bloom, S.R. & Polak, J.M. (1990). The endocrine gastrointestinal tract: tumors. In *Principles and Practice of Endocrinology and Metabolism*, ed. K.L. Becker, pp 1337–42. Philadelphia: Lippincott.

Grauer, A., Raue, F. & Gagel, R.F. (1990). Changing concepts in the management of hereditary and sporadic medullary thyroid carcinoma. *Endocrinol. Metab. Clin. North Am.* 19:613–35.

Lips, C.J.M., Landsvater, R.M., Hoppener, J.W.M., et al. (1994). Clinical screening as compared with DNA analysis in families with multiple endocrine neoplasia type 2A. *N. Engl. J. Med.* 331:828–32.

Mazzaferri, E.L. (1990). Thyroid cancer. In *Principles and Practice of Endocrinology and Metabolism*, ed. K.L. Becker, pp 319–31. Philadelphia: Lippincott.

Sizemore, G.W. (1990). Multiple endocrine neoplasia. In *Principles and Practice of Endocrinology and Metabolism*, ed. K.L. Becker, pp 1393–400. Philadelphia: Lippincott.

Pancreatic disease and carcinoma

Ammann, R.W. (1990). Chronic pancreatitis in the elderly. *Gastroenterol. Clin. North Am.* 19:905–14.

Perez, M.M., Newcomer, A.D., Moertel, C.G., Go, V.L. & Dimagno, E.P. (1983). Assessment of weight loss, food intake, fat metabolism, malabsorption, and treatment of pancreatic insufficiency in pancreatic cancer. *Cancer* 52:346–52.

Reber, H.A. (1987). Chronic pancreatitis. In *Surgical Diseases of the Pancreas*, ed. J.M. Howard, G.L. Jordan & H.A. Reber, pp. 475–95. Philadelphia: Lea & Febiger.

Radiation enteritis

Fenoglio-Preiser, C.M., Lantz, P.E., Davis, M., Listrom, M.B. & Rilke, F.O. (1989). The non-neoplastic large intestine. In *Gastrointestinal Pathology. An Atlas and Text*, ed. C.M. Fenoglio-Preiser, pp. 619–725. New York: Raven Press.

Fenoglio-Preiser, C.M., Lantz, P.E., Davis, M., Listrom, M.B. & Rilke, F.O. (1989). The non-neoplastic small intestine. In *Gastrointestinal Pathology. An Atlas and Text*, ed. C.M. Fenoglio-Preiser, pp. 245–357. New York: Raven Press.

Somatostatinoma

Boden, G. & Shelmet, J.J. (1987). Gastrointestinal hormones and the carcinoid tumors and syndrome. In *Endocrinology and Metabolism*, 2nd edn, ed. P. Felig, J.D. Baxter, A.E. Broadus & L.A. Frohman, pp. 1629–62. New York: McGraw-Hill.

Rood, P.R. & Donowitz, M. (1991). Endocrine tumor–associated diarrhoea syndromes. In *Diarrhoeal Diseases*, ed. M. Field, pp. 397–411. New York: Elsevier.

Systemic mastocytosis

Debeuckelaere, S., Schoors, D.F. & Davis, G. (1991). Systemic mast cell disease: a review of the literature with specific focus on the gastrointestinal manifestations. *Acta. Clinica. Belg.* 46:226–32.

Wasserman, S.I. (1990). The endocrine mast cell. In *Principles and Practice of Endocrinology and Metabolism,* ed. K.L. Becker, pp 1321–5. Philadelphia: Lippincott.

VIPoma

Bloom, S.R. & Polak, J.M. (1990). The endocrine gastrointestinal tract: tumors. In *Principles and Practice of Endocrinology and Metabolism,* ed. K.L. Becker, pp 1337–42. Philadelphia: Lippincott.

O'Dorisio, T.M., Mekhjian, H.S. & Gaginella, T.S. (1989). Medical therapy of VIPomas. *Endocrinol. Metab. Clin. North Am.* **18:**545–56.

Rambaud, J-C., Hautefenille, M., Ruskone, A. & Jacquenod, P. (1986). Diarrhoea due to circulating agents. *Clin. Gastroenterol.* **15:**603–29.

Rood, R.P., de Lellis, R.A., Dayal, Y. & Donowitz, M. (1988). Pancreatic cholera syndrome due to a vasoactive intestinal polypeptide-producing tumor: further insights into the pathophysiology. *Gastroenterol.* **94:**813–8.

Part IV
Constipation

16 Constipation: aetiology and diagnosis

Michael C. Woodward

Constipation is a common complaint amongst older people, and a frequent concern for their health care providers in hospital, long-term care setting, clinics and general practice. Physician visits for constipation increase markedly for patients over 60 years old, and laxative use also increases with age. Around 30 per cent of older Australians use laxatives regularly, including 40 per cent of females over the age of 80. To understand this major health concern we need to examine the effects of age in the physiology of bowel function, the causes of constipation and diagnostic approaches.

Definition

Constipation can be defined as:

- less than three bowel actions per week
- reduced faecal volume
- harder faecal consistency
- straining on more than 25 per cent of occasions
- excess faeces on rectal examination or abdominal x-ray

It is often more helpful to consider constipation as being possibly present when there is a change in one of these features in the individual. Older persons who have a regular bowel action each morning, passed with little straining, will appropriately consider themselves to be constipated if this suddenly changes to once every two days with straining every fourth occasion, even though this falls outside of the strict definition of constipation. Conversely, one needs to seek specific details of a self report of constipation before accepting this as the diagnosis.

Epidemiology

Much of the research on frequency of constipation is based on patient self report, which may be influenced by numerous factors including the perceived benefits of purgation, an imprecise perception of what is constipation, a life-long concern with bowel function, and anxiety or depression exaggerating the perception of constipation. It has been shown that older people often underestimate the frequency of their bowel actions.

Several studies of community-dwelling older people have shown complaints of constipation to be present in 30 to 60 per cent of the populations studied. A study of day-hospital attendees found the prevalence of self-reported constipation to be 55 per cent. There are no studies with adequate methodology in long-term care residents, but those published put the prevalence at around 60 to 70 per cent.

Despite this high self-reported prevalence, numerous studies show no reduction of bowel action frequency with normal aging; 94 to 99 per cent of both young and older community-dwelling individuals have three or more bowel actions per week. This suggests older people do overreport constipation or, alternatively, that individual changes in bowel action pattern, even within the normal range, are more common in older people. In support of this overreporting, 52 to 65 per cent of older people who complain of constipation report having bowel actions at least once daily and only 2–7 per cent report two or less bowel movements a week. Laxative use does not correlate with the frequency of bowel movements, suggesting older people do not maintain normal bowel actions (and thus actually correctly considering themselves constipated) with laxatives. Most interestingly, placebo treatments alone cure 60 per cent of those self-reporting constipation, and 55 per cent of habitual laxative users have normal bowel actions off laxatives.

Bowel function in older people

Three to four times a day part of the caecal contents pass through the colon to the rectum, propelled by strong contractions, known as mass peristalsis. This is to be distinguished from the smaller peristaltic stripping waves used to mix the colonic contents and facilitate water and electrolyte reabsorption. Food stimulates mass peristalsis hormonally – the gastrocolic reflex.

The rectal distension arising from this mass peristalsis stimulates the defaecation reflex, centred in the sacral cord. This can be inhibited by higher (medullary and cortical) centres so the rectum relaxes and the process ceases. If not inhibited, defaecation occurs as a coordinated movement of both voluntary and involuntary muscles. The sensation of rectal distension is first associated with increasing contraction of the external anal sphincter, then internal anal sphincter relaxation. This allows 'sampling' of the rectal contents, to distinguish between solid, liquid and gas. The external sphincter remains contracted until it is voluntarily relaxed – then defaecation occurs.

The amount of faeces passed varies; sometimes the whole left colon empties, sometimes only part of the rectum. A self-reported, or observer-reported 'good' bowel action does not mean the passage of all, or even the majority, of the stored faecal material.

Normal aging does not prolong colonic transit time, but it may be prolonged in unwell older people, especially those bed-bound and in long-term care, and in those who are indeed constipated. Slower transit in unwell older people may result from reduced oral intake, immobility or medications.

Internal anal sphincter tone is probably not greatly affected by aging, or illness, or in those with constipation. External anal sphincter tone is reduced by both aging and illness, and more so in those with constipation. Rectal tone is unaffected by normal aging, and studies on those with constipation or chronic illness yield varying results. Rectal sensation is also unaffected by normal aging, but is reduced by illness or chronic constipation.

Electrophysiological studies have shown a diminished sigmoid motor response to colonic stimulation in constipated older people, but this effective denervation may be due to previous laxative use. Normal aging does not appear to affect the motor response. One study has shown a reduced amplitude of inhibitory junction potentials with age, suggesting a predisposition to segmental motor incoordination and functional partial bowel obstruction.

Hormonal and receptor influences on bowel function may be altered with aging. Increased endorphin binding in older people's colons has been demonstrated, which could inhibit motility and increase resting anal tone. Interestingly, naloxone given to nursing-home residents with constipation did increase stool output and reduce symptoms of constipation. There is little or no change in the levels of gut neuropeptides with aging.

Types of constipation

There is some value in dividing constipation into two subtypes. In one, there is increased rectal tone and reduced compliance, causing the patient to complain of difficult passage of hard faecal pellets. In the second, called 'rectal dyschezia', there is reduced rectal tone, a variable degree of rectal dilatation, impaired rectal sensation and a higher volume of rectal distension required to induce reflex relaxation of the internal anal sphincter. Patients affected by this second type present more often with faecal impaction, which they may be unaware of. This second type may be due to diminished parasympathetic outflow from the sacral cord, due to conditions such as ischaemia and spinal stenosis.

Causes of constipation

These causes of constipation are summarized below:

- misperception
- voluntary
- dietary – these include: reduced food intake; poor dentition; other

- immobility – due to: illness; pain; bed rest; lack of exercise
- geography, e.g. toilet poorly designed, lack of privacy, unable to reach toilet
- drugs – see below
- metabolic or endocrine, including: hypercalcaemia, hypothyroidism
- gut lesions, as a result of obstruction, carcinoma, volvulus, ischaemia, radiation, aganglionosis (primary and acquired, e.g. laxatives), and diverticular disease
- anal lesions, including fissures, haemorrhoids
- neurogenic, for example spinal cord lesions (e.g. multiple sclerosis), Parkinson's disease, diabetes mellitus, strokes
- depression
- dementia.

Medications that cause constipation include narcotics (codeine, pethidine, morphine (variably)); anticholinergics; antispasmodics (e.g. diphenoxylate); antidepressants (e.g. imipramine); antipsychotics (e.g. chlorpromazine); antiparkinsonian medications (e.g. benztropine); anion-containing agents such as iron, aluminium (antacids, sucralfate), and calcium; neurally active agents such as antihypertensives (e.g. alpha methyl dopa), calcium channel blockers (e.g. verapamil), and anticonvulsants (e.g. phenytoin); and diuretics.

Constipation has numerous causes, and multiple causes are often present in older people. The assessment must include a detailed history, examination and appropriate investigations.

Misperception is not uncommon, as already discussed. Voluntary constipation may occur on long journeys, or when toilet facilities are inadequate or difficult to access. Food and fluid intake may be reduced due to illness or simply to lack of available food. Although there is no prospective evidence that reducing fluid intake causes constipation, it is clinically reasonable. Older people are prone to dehydration due to reduced thirst sensation and impaired fluid homeostasis. Many older people prefer to avoid high-fibre foods, or may not be offered such foods (for example, in hospital). There is actually little clinical evidence that fibre intake correlates with true constipation. Very high fibre intake clearly causes frequent, bulky, soft bowel actions. One community study showed no reduction in the symptoms of constipation with a higher fibre diet, but four nonrandomized nursing-home studies showed the addition of bran reduced laxative use.

Poor mobility is common, particularly when an older person is unwell, and exercise stimulates mass peristalsis – one study showed that simply assuming an upright position reduced enema use in bedridden older people. Toilet facilities available to older people are often substandard. One study on toilet facilities in a teaching hospital showed that none met British Standards Association recommendations. The facilities were worse on the geriatric medicine wards, with no signposting or labelling, small (1.5 x 0.9 m) size, and a narrow (0.7 m) door that disallowed frame or wheelchair access. In one geriatric medicine ward, all the toilets had been closed off and only commodes were available.

Multiple medications increase the risk of constipation, and are more commonly prescribed to older people than younger people. Again, however, there are few prospective studies but numerous case reports. Some drugs which theoretically should cause constipation do not seem to – nonsteroidal anti-inflammatory drugs (prostaglandin inhibition) and angiotensin-converting enzyme inhibitors (smooth muscle relaxation) are examples.

Hypokalaemia causes neuronal dysfunction that reduces acetylcholine stimulation of gut smooth muscle, prolonging gut transit time. Hypercalcaemia causes conduction delay within extrinsic and intrinsic innervation of the gut. Hypothyroidism may cause constipation via myxoedematous oedema of the gut wall.

The most serious cause of constipation is a bowel tumour, and this must be suspected when no other cause is apparent or if the constipation persists. Volvulus may be painless in older people, and can have serious consequences if not rapidly detected. Ischaemic colitis is more common with age, and may be associated with atrial fibrillation. Rarely, primary aganglionosis presents in older age – more commonly, older age aganglionosis is associated with long-term laxative use. Diverticular disease may be a consequence of high colonic pressures associated with constipation, and may itself cause constipation. Anal fissures and haemorrhoids may cause a voluntary constipation due to pain on defaecation.

Spinal cord lesions in older people are caused more commonly by multiple sclerosis, spinal cord stenosis, ischaemia, tumours, infections and trauma (the latter sometimes related to osteoporotic vertebral crush fractures).

Patients with Parkinson's disease may suffer greatly from constipation as a result of prolonged transit throughout the entire gut, independent of age, immobility or anticholinergic use, and anal sphincter dysfunction. Diabetes mellitus is also a risk factor, due perhaps to associated autonomic neuropathy. Strokes may cause constipation by weakness of the abdominal and pelvic muscles and hypomotility of the large bowel, and pontine damage may induce altered behavioural responses to a full rectum.

Depression and dementia predispose to rectal impaction, independently of other associated features such as immobility, dehydration and medication exposure. The mechanism may be partly through ignoring the urge to defaecate. Psychological distress may also increase the self reporting of constipation; indeed from some older people the complaint of constipation may simply mean the person feels unwell.

As with many other illnesses in older people constipation often has multiple causes, and a search for the aetiology should not cease because one cause has been found.

Diagnosis

It is important to establish whether the constipation is genuine – details about stool frequency, consistency, volume and straining will often achieve this but sometimes a stool chart needs to be kept for a week or two. The duration of constipation and past episodes should be noted.

The history must also include details of past anorectal disease or surgery, other illnesses and drugs taken. Previous and current laxative use, including over-the-counter preparations (which may not be recognized by the patient as a medication), needs to be documented. Diet and fluid intake, particularly recent changes, should be noted. The toilet facilities should be noted. Mobility and exercises should be enquired into.

Associated features, such as faecal and urinary incontinence, diarrhoea, abdominal or perianal pain, bleeding and constitutional symptoms (weight loss, fever, confusion), should be sought.

The physical examination should note hydration, weight loss, cognition and mood. A detailed abdominal examination is essential, searching for palpable faeces, colonic dilatation, other masses and a palpable bladder. The absence of palpable faeces does not exclude the diagnosis of constipation.

Rectal examination must be performed. Faecal impaction may be detected this way, and has an important bearing on management. Other rectal masses, blood, perianal pathology and anal tone and sensation should be noted. Perineal and saddle sensation can also be assessed at this stage.

Neurological examination for evidence of a spinal cord lesion, autonomic or other neuropathy should be performed. Endocrine examination should search for signs of hypothyroidism and hypercalcaemia.

Investigations are not always necessary. An abdominal x-ray is usually necessary if the rectal examination is unremarkable, to exclude high faecal impaction. The correlation between the rectal examination and abdominal x-ray is poor, with faecal impaction often shown with only one of these.

If colonic pathology is suspected in history or examination, colonoscopy or barium enema is indicated. The preparation for these not infrequently is a definitive cure of the constipation!

Other investigations more commonly indicated include electrolytes, calcium, haemoglobin and thyroid function. Tests rarely required include tumour markers, neurological imaging and abdominal ultrasound.

Constipation is a common complaint of older people, but care should be taken before assuming it is actually present. There are changes in large bowel and anal function found in unwell or constipated older people, but few with normal aging.

Constipation has numerous causes, and multiple causes are often present in older people. The assessment must include a detailed history, examination and appropriate investigations.

BIBLIOGRAPHY AND FURTHER READING

Harari, D., Gurwitz, J.H. & Minaker, K.L. (1993). Constipation in the elderly. *J. Am. Geriatr. Soc.* 41:1130–40.

Wald, A. (1990). Constipation and fecal incontinence in the elderly. *Gastroenterol. Clin. North Am.* 19:405–18.

Wald, A. (1993). Constipation in elderly patients. Pathogenesis and management. *Drugs Aging* 3:220–31.

Whitehead, W.E., Drinkwater, D., Cheskin, L.J., Heller, B.R. & Schuster, M.M. (1989). Constipation in the elderly living at home. Definition, prevalence, and relationship to lifestyle and health status. *J. Am. Geriatr. Soc.* 37:423–9.

Wrenn, K. (1989). Fecal impaction. *N. Engl. J. Med.* 321:658–62.

 Constipation: issues of management

Michael C. Woodward

Complications

Constipation is not a benign condition. The many possible complications include: faecal impaction, faecal incontinence, urinary incontinence, urinary retention, anorectal disorders (e.g. prolapse, fissures, haemorrhoids), rectal distension, bowel obstruction, volvulus, idiopathic megacolon, arrhythmias, vasovagal episodes, transient ischaemic attacks, angina, myocardial infarction, pulmonary embolism, anorexia, nausea, delirium, distress and laxative abuse.

Faecal impaction can be hard or soft. The major complication of this is faecal incontinence (see Chapter 6), which is due to the impacted faeces irritating the adjacent mucosa and causing mucus and fluid secretion, rather than overflow of more proximal faeces. The anal sphincter remains well contracted even in the presence of chronic faecal impaction, but this is inadequate to retain the fluid products of the mucosal irritation.

Urinary incontinence can occur from irritation to the bladder outlet by impacted faeces, or as overflow from urinary retention caused by faecal obstruction to bladder emptying. Rectal prolapse is more often worsened but may be caused by impaction. Anal fissures can both cause and be a consequence of constipation. Haemorrhoids, haemorrhoidal bleeding and even anaemia can be caused or worsened by constipation.

Bowel obstruction from faecal impaction or a faecolith is uncommon but does occur. Idiopathic megacolon may be caused by laxatives or constipation. It may present as progressive, painless abdominal swelling often in bed-ridden residents of long-term care institutions. The main danger is volvulus, which is not infrequently fatal.

Constipation can induce anorexia, nausea and vomiting that may be poorly tolerated by an older person who is afflicted by other illnesses. Delirium may be solely caused by constipation, but other causes should be sought. The cardiac and embolic complications of constipation are usually but not invariably associated with straining. A classical scenario is the postoperative patient who collapses while straining on the toilet.

Older people were raised in an era where infrequent bowel actions were perceived to cause systemic illness and autointoxication; constipation can therefore cause considerable distress.

Constipation requires prompt and appropriate management. This includes non-pharmacological and pharmacological approaches.

Nonpharmacological management of constipation

The approach to the older person complaining of constipation should include education about normal bowel habit and the importance of adequate fibre, fluid and exercise.

Dietary fibre consists of soluble and insoluble fibre. Soluble fibre intake is associated with lowering serum lipids and improving diabetic control but has a minimal effect in resolving constipation since stool weight is not significantly increased. Examples of soluble fibre are: pears, apples, peas, lentils and oats. Insoluble fibres occur in wheat brans, wheat and barley. The beneficial effects which relieve constipation are increasing stool bulk, accelerating intestinal transit and reducing colonic pressure.

Between 30 and 35 grams of fibre per day is adequate. Sources of dietary fibre include breakfast cereals (but care should be exercised because some are very low, even mueslis and others whose marketing suggests otherwise), other grain products, fruit and vegetables. These should be discussed with the older patient who may have poor knowledge of fibre, reflecting dietary habits earlier this century. High fibre diets should be avoided if there is colonic dilatation or faecal impaction.

An adequate fluid intake is around 1500 ml/day – many older people do not drink this much, and more may be required in warmer weather or for those on diuretics. Exercise needs to be commenced cautiously, but even minimal levels may improve bowel function.

Improved toilet habits may resolve constipation. There should be adequate privacy, time and comfort. This is particularly important in institutional settings. The toilet should be accessible. Generally, the most successful time to use the toilet is after breakfast, when the gastrocolic reflex is active, but individuals vary. Leg elevation may improve bowel function by helping the use of weakened abdominal and pelvic floor muscles.

Laxative use should be stopped whenever possible, particularly where there is no constipation present or the condition resolves. Other medications should be carefully reviewed and those possibly contributing to constipation should be stopped, where practical.

Underlying causes should be treated – particularly painful haemorrhoids and fissures. Even if the underlying condition cannot be cured, other nonpharmacological initiatives may lead to improvement.

Laxatives: issues

Laxative use and abuse may begin with a minor episode of constipation, a misperception of constipation or merely concern about the risk of constipation. They are not infrequently continued at home after being commenced in hospital, establishing a habit of usage that may persist. Whatever the cause, laxatives are the second most commonly consumed over-the-counter medication, with 30 per cent of older people using them at least weekly, as noted in Chapter 19. Studies have demonstrated laxatives prescribed to 76 per cent of hospitalized older people and 74 per cent of nursing home residents. However, 20 to 30 per cent of laxative users do not consider themselves to be constipated, and in one study 77.5 per cent of regular users had never gone more than three days without a bowel action.

Laxatives are associated with damage to the myenteric plexus, colonic hypomotility and dilatation (cathartic colon). Melanosis coli has also been associated with several laxatives but itself is probably benign. Other complications of laxative use include fluid and electrolyte depletion, alkalosis, hypocalcaemia and malabsorption. Clearly, they should be used cautiously, and preferably only short term.

There have been few advances in laxatives over the last 50 years – this is relatively unique in therapeutics. Additionally, there have been few well controlled comparative trials. The high placebo response rate has been noted. In one recent randomized double blind crossover study comparing senna and fibre with lactulose, lactulose was less effective than the cheaper regime. Clearly more such studies are needed.

Laxatives: use

Where laxatives are deemed necessary, they should be used along with the nonpharmacological approaches discussed above. The laxatives and enemas in common use are summarized below:

- bulking agents, including bran, ispaghula, sterculia, psyllium and other fibres
- stool softeners, e.g. docusate and bisacodyl
- colonic stimulants, such as senna and castor oil
- osmotic agents, e.g. lactulose, polyethylene glycol and sorbitol
- lubricants, e.g. paraffin
- secretagogues, e.g. phenolphthalein
- saline laxatives, such as magnesium sulphate, magnesium phosphate and magnesium citrate

- enemas and suppositories, including soap and water, phosphate, sodium salts or sorbitol, glycerol, bisacodyl.

Bulking agents

Bulking agents absorb water, increasing stool bulk and water content. This increases colonic motility. Bacterial fermentation can cause bloating and flatulence, particularly with bran and the natural fibres. If they are used with inadequate water there is a risk of impaction.

Bran is a pentose-containing polysaccharide that can be mixed with or incorporated into breakfast cereals, or baked into bread and cakes. Use has been associated with iron malabsorption.

The other agents are produced as powders requiring reconstitution or in a granular form that should be variously swallowed whole or sprinkled on food. These agents do not cause malabsorption of iron, fat soluble vitamins or digoxin. Psyllium, the most expensive, also lowers serum cholesterol but some feel it is the least effective of the bulking agents.

Stool softeners

Docusate sodium is an anionic detergent that lowers stool surface tension, allowing water to penetrate and soften the stool. It also causes colonic mucosal irritation. Between 50 and 120 mg/day is sufficient, but it must be used with adequate water. The softer stool may increase the risk of faecal incontinence. As less straining is required, this may be useful to patients with angina, haemorrhoids and where there is a risk of pulmonary embolism.

Bisacodyl probably acts more as a stool softener than a colonic stimulant. It is often used as a preparative for radiological imaging.

Colonic stimulants

Senna is a glycoside that is hydrolysed by colonic bacteria into absorbable anthroquinones that directly stimulate the myenteric plexus to increase colonic motility. It also alters electrolyte transport and increases intraluminal fluids. It is available as tablets, granules or in combination with other products such as fruit or docusate. Senna generally works within 12 hours, but this may be prolonged in older patients, in whom it may take 10 weeks of daily dosing to achieve a regular bowel habit. Bedtime use reduces the risk of nocturnal faecal incontinence.

Castor oil is associated with a high risk of adverse effects such as malabsorption and dehydration, and is not recommended for use in older people.

All stimulant laxatives can cause malabsorption of fats and electrolytes, so their use should be limited. However, maintenance therapy with senna two or three times a week may be needed in chronically ill older people with prolonged bowel transit time. Other adverse effects of these agents include cramping and diarrhoea.

Osmotic agents

Lactulose is a nonabsorbable disaccharide which is broken down in the colon by lactobacilli into smaller osmotically active organic acids which attract water into the lumen. This increases stool softness and shortens colonic transit time.

Sorbitol has a similar action. Polyethylene glycol is a more potent hyperosmolar laxative currently used in bowel preparation for colonoscopy, barium enema and surgery. However, the required volume of two litres, usually consumed over a few hours, may be poorly tolerated by older people. It is of proven benefit for the relief of colonic impaction.

Lubricants

Paraffin is a commonly consumed laxative in Australia, often combined with phenolphthalein. The lubricated faeces are more easily passed, but faecal incontinence and pruritus ani may occur. Other adverse effects include lipoid pneumonia, granulomatous hepatitis and malabsorption of fat soluble vitamins. It is contraindicated where there is a risk of aspiration. Indeed, it is far from an ideal laxative in older people and its use should be discouraged.

Secretagogues

Phenolphthalein is an enterotoxin not unlike cholera toxin, causing the pumping of fluid and electrolytes into the lumen. It has a long duration of action and can cause skin reactions. Its use is probably best avoided in older people.

Saline laxatives

These draw fluid osmotically into the small bowel lumen. Magnesium hydroxide also stimulates the release of the prokinetic hormone cholecystokinin. They have a rapid onset of action, inducing evacuation usually within three hours. They may cause abdominal cramping, dehydration and faecal incontinence of the watery stools. Hypermagnesaemia is a risk, especially if there is renal insufficiency. They are thus far from ideal in older people, but remain popular.

Enemas and suppositories

Enemas induce evacuation by causing rectal distension and mucosal irritation by small osmotically active molecules. They also have a lavage effect. They can damage the rectal mucosa especially if used repeatedly and must be administered carefully. The most common explanation of a poor result is inadequate administration. Hyperphosphataemia has been associated with phosphate enemas.

Glycerol suppositories are hyperosmolar and soften the stool. Bisacodyl suppositories are locally active and poorly absorbed. Both are most useful for rectal dyschezia but can cause rectal irritation.

Management of constipation

It is essential to first establish whether the person is not actually constipated, at high risk of becoming constipated, well and acutely constipated, unwell and acutely constipated or chronically constipated. If the person is constipated, faecal impaction *must* be sought as this requires treatment first, and oral therapy may be dangerous in the presence of untreated faecal impaction.

Faecal impaction may respond to enemas or suppositories. If hard impaction fails to respond, or the volume is so large that response to enemas and suppositories is unlikely, manual disimpaction will be needed. This can be very uncomfortable and an anaesthetic gel is usually needed. Repeated manual disimpaction may be required, over several days. Rarely, surgical disimpaction is needed. Once enemas or suppositories are working, they should be given once or twice daily until rectal examination and abdominal x-ray show clearance. If colonic faecal loading persists, in the absence of obstruction, polyethylene glycol is useful. Once the impaction has resolved, oral laxatives are usually required for some time. Colonic neoplasm must be considered if impaction remains resistant or recurs.

For all other types of constipation, nonpharmacological management should be initiated. The exception is where impaction or colonic dilatation preclude the initial use of increased dietary fibre.

High risk situations such as surgery or the commencement of narcotic analgesia warrant consideration of a short course of a laxative. A stimulant such as senna, up to one tablet three times a day, is appropriate.

In otherwise well, acutely constipated older people, a hierarchical approach is reasonable, commencing with nonpharmacological management that may take a few days to work. If this fails, bulking agents followed by senna, sorbitol or docusate should be used. If straining is predominant, a suppository may be useful, often as sole therapy.

In frail or unwell, acutely constipated older people, again commence with nonpharmacological management. Bulking agents are more likely to be contraindicated in this population, due to poor fluid intake or colonic dilatation. Senna, sorbitol or docusate, often in combination with a suppository, should be used if the other approaches fail or are contraindicated. The person should be closely monitored for the development of faecal impaction.

Chronic constipation can be difficult to treat, particularly if associated with long-term laxative use. Colonic dilatation is more likely and initial use of dietary fibre or bulking agents is thus likely to be inappropriate. Prolonged use of enemas or polyethylene glycol may be needed to treat impaction. Once this has resolved, sorbitol or lactulose may be required to maintain colonic transit. If other laxatives have been used long term they may need to be continued initially, then progressively weaned. Once the colon is not dilated or impacted, bulking agents can be introduced and may be required long term. The nonpharmacological approaches must be reinforced repeatedly. Missed underlying causes, such as hypothyroidism, should be considered if the condition recurs or remains refractory.

Nonpharmacological management is appropriate to both prevent and treat constipation. Despite few recent additions, there is an extensive array of pharmacological treatments, but all are associated with adverse effects, especially if used excessively. Some are safer in older people. Oral and rectal treatment should both be considered. Underlying pathology should be excluded when constipation is recurrent or refractory.

BIBLIOGRAPHY AND FURTHER READING

Castle, S.C. (1989). Constipation: endemic in the elderly? Gerontopathophysiology, evaluation and management. *Med. Clin. North Am.* **73**:1497–509.

Hope, A.K. & Down, E.C. (1986). Dietary fibre and fluid in the control of constipation in a nursing home population. *Med. J. Aust.* **144**:306–7.

Smith, R.G. & Lewis, S. (1990). The relationship between digital rectal examination and abdominal radiographs in elderly patients. *Age Ageing* **19**:142–3.

Wald, A. (1993). Constipation in elderly patients. Pathogenesis and management. *Drugs Aging* **3**:220–31.

Wrenn, K. (1989). Fecal impaction. *N. Engl. J. Med.* **321**:658–62.

Part V

Perspectives of altered bowel function

18   Issues of nutrition

Ian Darnton-Hill, Seppo K. Suomela and N.V.K. Nair

Introduction

The relatively rapid and universal increase in longevity has been attributed, amongst other things, to an improvement in nutrition in both childhood and later life. The increasing attention being paid to nutrition in hospital patients, institutionalized elderly and those with risk factors for the chronic noncommunicable diseases, has also played a role.

One of the factors involved in the nutritional consequences of disease is that older people generally have a reduced safety margin in times of nutritional stress. Nutrient stores are often less, intake sometimes marginal and utilization less efficient. Consequently, the onset of disease, or a chronic state, both of which can be presenting forms of diarrhoea, can adversely affect the nutritional status of the elderly patient.

A reduction in the nutritional status can negatively affect the immune state of the elderly person, leading to an increase in infections, or a reduction in the ability to fight pre-existing gastrointestinal infection. This may therefore initiate a cycle in which the poor nutritional state leads to sustained disease which, in turn, leads to further impairment of nutrition. In a study in the USA which looked at the characteristics related to elderly persons not eating for one or more days, diarrhoea itself was one factor involved.

In children the effect of diarrhoea on nutritional status depends upon the level of energy (calorie) intake, just as the negative effect of an inadequate energy intake on nutritional status depends on the severity and duration of diarrhoea. In children, when the nutritional status is not compromised by an inadequate energy intake, diarrhoea has a minimal negative effect on growth, as has been observed among well nourished children in the USA. It may be possible to extrapolate this finding to the elderly with its implications for management. Similarities in terms of interaction between nutrition and immune function in infants and the elderly have been identified. Both have less than optimal immune responses and a high risk of developing infections and, in both, dietary factors are important.

Nutrition in the elderly

This can be considered under three headings: (*a*) nutritional status of elderly people; (*b*) factors, including diarrhoea, likely to lead to malnutrition; and (*c*) specific nutrients at risk in the elderly.

Nutritional status

The significance of nutrition in aging is that many physiological functions decline progressively throughout adult life, such as demineralization of the skeleton, host immunity and food intake in general. Lastly, although this will not be discussed, aging is associated with the emergence of the chronic diseases, including those of nutritional aetiology.

Changes in body composition occur throughout adult life with a continuous decline in lean body mass, which tends to accelerate in later life and be greater in males. In addition to loss of active tissue mass, reduction occurs in the function of many organs and tissues, e.g. cellular enzymes for men between 30 and 80 years of age fall by 15 per cent; resting cardiac output by 30 per cent; and renal blood flow by 50 per cent.

Metabolic functions are progressively altered with aging. The rates of synthesis and breakdown of protein, expressed as 'per kilogram body weight', are significantly lower in older people of both sexes. Total body protein synthesis, body mass and bone mineralization decrease, while the proportion of body fat increases.

In the gastrointestinal tract the physiological changes of aging have only limited effects on nutritional status and well being of the elderly.

Immunological function is depressed by aging and by malnutrition, although the actual relationship is unclear and differs from one individual to the next. Elderly patients often develop deficiencies in host defences that may predispose to infectious diarrhoea (see Chapters 1 and 2), although 25 per cent of elderly individuals have immune responses as vigorous as those of young adults.

Tissue avidity for some nutrients appears to be reduced by aging and nutrient uptake decreases, e.g. zinc. There is evidence of a decrease in the utilization of polyglutamate forms of folacin from foods, although synthetic folic acid is well absorbed at all ages. There is no evidence that the absorption of other B vitamins is affected.

There is still controversy regarding the role of nutritional factors in age-related bone mineral loss involving calcium intake, the role of high amounts of protein in the diet and the role of vitamin D. The relationship between physical activity, satiety and nutritional status is complex and not well understood. The loss of acuity of sweet and salt tastes with advancing age is yet another factor that affects dietary intake and, hence, nutritional status.

Malnutrition in the elderly is described in both industrialized and developed countries, particularly in the hospitalized and institutionalized elderly and those with poor social circumstances. There are relatively few data on the nutritional status of ambulatory, institutionalized elderly. One study in the USA concluded that 'malnutrition, both with and without concomitant major co-morbid diseases, is relatively frequent among elderly ambulatory patients and that a specific nutritional diagnosis is not made in many cases'. However, in this biased sample, which had received care from a medical faculty practice, only 3.25 per cent were classified as malnourished.

In Australia early studies showed low intakes of vitamins C and A and iron, with biochemical values suggesting that nutrient inadequacy was not uncommon but that clinical manifestations of deficiency were rare. When community-based and institutionalized elderly persons in the Melbourne area were compared, plasma vitamin C, folate, albumin and zinc levels were lower in the institutionalized subjects. In other studies dietary intakes of zinc, vitamin D, vitamin E, vitamin B_6, total folate, calcium and dietary fibre were low when compared with the recommended intakes. This does not, of course, necessarily mean that these subjects were clinically malnourished.

Factors leading to malnutrition

Specific risk factors exist that identify elderly individuals who are especially likely to be malnourished. For example, isolation and various socioeconomic difficulties can lead to markedly changed patterns of eating, as can problems with dentition. A British study reported that low intakes of vitamin C by elderly males and low serum pyridoxine levels in elderly females were predictive of early mortality.

An important cause of malnutrition in the elderly is pharmaceuticals. Hypertensive drugs adversely influence potassium and magnesium status, antibiotics affect intestinal absorption and hypnotics affect nutritional intake behaviour.

For the elderly living in the community, the degree of dependence is important. The more dependent the elderly are on being fed by others, the greater the risk of malnutrition.

The study referred to earlier regarding the characteristics of the elderly not eating for one or more days, implicated, in addition to diarrhoea, other factors such as ethnicity, location, receipt of Medicaid (generally an indicator of socioeconomic status), living alone, health problems, mobility, age greater than 80 years, cancer, nausea, difficulty swallowing, loss of appetite and receiving food from a food pantry. The finding that living alone was positively related to not eating among men, but not among women, has also been reported with national US data and in other studies.

Psychological, psychosocial and socioeconomic factors, such as depression and dementia, can be of great importance to the nutritional status of elderly people. Certain older people are particularly at risk of malnutrition: the physically isolated, those living alone (especially those recently bereaved), the socially isolated, those with sensory or mental impairment, those with chronic systemic disease, the very poor and the very old.

Food contamination or improper food handling, especially for those living alone and preparing food under less than ideal conditions, are also factors leading to possible gastrointestinal disease and which may in turn lead to malnutrition. Travel is yet another factor to be considered.

There is a progressive decrease in energy intake and, probably, requirements with age. One study showed a progressive decrease in average daily intake from 2700 kcal at 20–34 years to 2100 kcal at 75–90 years. One third of this fall (200 kcal) was accounted for by the reduction in basal energy metabolism consequent on reduced body cell mass, while the remaining 400 kcal were identified as the result of reduced activity. The sharp decline in the energy intake of the very old is often related to disability and chronic disease.

In most diets, as energy intakes fall there is a very strong likelihood that the intake of other nutrients will also fall. Nutrients that are identified as being at risk include iron, thiamine, riboflavin and nicotinic acid, with no evidence of a downward trend for calcium, vitamin A or vitamin C. The most common deficiency in the elderly in both developing and industrialized countries is iron which affects both resistance to infection and cognition. Protein inadequacy is likely with the diets consumed by many of the elderly and would thus contribute to increased susceptibility to infection.

Specific nutrients at risk in the elderly

Relying on clinical examination and laboratory tests, in conjunction with dietary history, the report of the Department of Health and Social Security on the elderly in the UK in 1979 concluded that 6 per cent of men and 5 per cent of women between 70 and 80 years of age, and 12 per cent of men and 8 per cent of women over 80 years of age, displayed one or more forms of malnutrition, which commonly consisted of protein-energy malnutrition and deficiencies of iron, vitamin B, folate, vitamin C or vitamin D.

Antihypertensive drugs can influence potassium and magnesium status. The clinical picture of magnesium deficiency is often coloured by superimposed hypocalcaemia and/or hypokalaemia. This can be aggravated by poor intake of potassium and magnesium due to anorexia and loop diuretics causing urinary magnesium loss. Magnesium depletion can be the result of severe diarrhoea and, as is the case for potassium, faecal magnesium excretion is related to the total water content of the stool.

The nutritional consequences of diarrhoea in the elderly

Given the situation outlined above, the consequences of diarrhoea in the elderly can be very severe. Important modifying factors are the pre-existing nutritional status, other concurrent illnesses, drug therapy, the severity and duration of the diarrhoea, and the appropriateness of the treatment given. The consequences will be discussed in terms of acute, persistent and chronic diarrhoea, but before that the interplay between aging, diarrhoea and malnutrition will be examined.

Aging, infection and malnutrition

Infections virtually always worsen nutritional status through a reduction of food intake and by increased internal and external metabolic losses; and, in the case of diarrhoea, through reduced absorption of nutrients. Diarrhoea in particular, and more so when accompanied by fever, can compromise energy and nutrient balance through three mechanisms: (*a*) reduced dietary intake; (*b*) increased faecal loss because of malabsorption of micronutrients and macronutrients, decreased intestinal transit time, and loss of nutrients into the gut; and (*c*) increased catabolism because of an acceleration in basal metabolic rate.

Diarrhoea is a symptom in some of the deficiency diseases which occurs only when the deficiency is quite severe, e.g. vitamin D deficiency, niacin deficiency and the intractable diarrhoea in the final stages of starvation.

Whilst diarrhoea is a well recognized problem in infants and young children, its impact in adults is less generally recognized. Hospital data of a sample from the McDonnell-Douglas Health Information System consisting of 4.06 million hospitalizations in 1985, was analysed. The analysis showed that, while children aged less than five years and adults aged 60 years or more each comprised one quarter of hospitalizations involving gastroenteritis, the older group represented 85 per cent of diarrhoea deaths. The data concluded that gastroenteritis is a large, underemphasized public health problem in the elderly, among whom the case:fatality ratio is higher than in children.

In a review of national mortality data compiled by the National Center for Health Statistics, consisting of information from all death certificates filed in the United States, it was found that the majority of diarrhoea deaths occurred among the elderly (older than 74 years, 51 per cent), followed by adults 55 to 74 years of age (27 per cent) and young children (<5 years, 11 per cent). The high morbidity in the elderly was due to increased susceptibility to dehydration, waning immunity and frequent institutionalization.

A death for which diarrhoea was listed as an immediate or underlying cause was considered a 'diarrhoeal death' and included in the analysis. However, some of the so-called unrelated conditions, e.g. cardiovascular diseases, make the elderly particularly susceptible to the complications of diarrhoea, such as electrolyte imbalance, dehydration and shock, and the figures may underestimate the real impact of diarrhoea in elderly mortality. Some other diseases more commonly seen in old age can also be associated with diarrhoea, e.g. a minority of postgastrectomy patients and when there is involvement of autonomic nerves in diabetes causing nocturnal diarrhoea.

Malnutrition is usually a complex syndrome of multiple nutrient deficiencies. Even moderate deficiencies of pyridoxine, folic acid, vitamin A, vitamin C and vitamin E can all result in impaired cell-mediated immunity and reduced antibody responses. Zinc deficiency is associated with lymphoid atrophy, slower cutaneous delayed hypersensitivity responses and homograft rejection and low thymic hormone activity. In general terms, immune responses decline in old age. As immunological vigour declines, the incidence of infections, cancer, immune complex disease, autoimmune disorders and amyloidosis increases.

Acute diarrhoea

Age has been found to be the single most important determinant of death subsequent to hospitalization involving gastroenteritis. Gastroenteritis deaths in the elderly are more likely to be associated with less severe disease (short hospitalizations, fewer complications and higher socioeconomic status) compared with gastrointestinal deaths in younger patients. This suggests greater frailty with advancing age and perhaps less resistance due to existing nutritional status.

In diarrhoea or vomiting large volumes of water may be lost with resultant dehydration. The normal small loss of water in the faeces is the balance of large exchanges taking place in the intestines (up to 8 litres of fluid or more per day). The greater part of the sodium and potassium entering the gut is absorbed and only about 150 ml of water, 5 mmol of sodium and 10 mmol of potassium lost in the faeces daily. The losses increase when absorption is impaired by diarrhoea. In the extreme case of cholera, absorption virtually ceases. The results are dramatic in terms of outflow of fluids almost isotonic with plasma, and large amounts of sodium and potassium.

Persistent and chronic diarrhoea

The elderly at greatest risk of death due to diarrhoea in hospital have, amongst other factors, more complications and longer hospital stays. These observations suggest the presence of other chronic diseases and/or nosocomial infections. Persistent diarrhoea is defined by the World Health Organization as diarrhoea that starts acutely but is of unusually long duration (at least 14 days). Chronic diarrhoea, on the other hand, is recurrent or long-lasting diarrhoea due usually to non-infectious causes, such as coeliac disease (see Chapter 11).

However, in a large study in the USA, it was not possible to distinguish the elderly cases with diarrhoea present at admission (i.e. community acquired) from those occurring in the hospital (nosocomial). Nor could acute diarrhoea be distinguished from persistent or chronic diarrhoea (as defined by that lasting more than two weeks), suggesting that any effects on mortality, at least, form part of a continuum.

In terms of management, the cumulative effects of mild ongoing diarrhoea are less obvious. Symptoms arising from depletion, especially of potassium, are easily overlooked. Magnesium deficiency may occur with prolonged diarrhoea from any cause.

In the malabsorption syndrome, lack of digestive secretions or a mucosal injury of the small intestine impair absorption of nutrients. Loss of weight and nutrient malabsorption occur. Anaemia is usually present due to impaired absorption of iron and folic acid. Nutritional glossitis, angular stomatitis and peripheral neuropathy can arise from deficiency of the B group vitamins, the first two commonly in early cases of malabsorption and the latter usually only in long-standing cases. Prolonged failure of calcium absorption may lead to evidence of osteomalacia and to tetany. Haemorrhages attributable to vitamin K may be present. Vitamin A deficiency from prolonged diarrhoea is rare.

Many elderly patients with malabsorption do not have pronounced symptoms and present with weight loss of unknown aetiology, persistent failure to gain weight after intercurrent illness, subclinical vitamin B_{12} deficiency, low serum folate determinations, nonspecific gastrointestinal symptoms, advanced osteopenia or hypoprothrombinaemia.

Tropical sprue (see Chapter 9) may present with the features of sore mouth and steatorrhoea, and the second or deficiency stage is punctuated by signs of undernutrition and vitamin deficiency, such as glossitis or stomatitis. In addition to defective absorption of fat, which is the feature most readily recognized, the absorption of water, electrolytes, glucose, vitamins and minerals is also impaired.

Malabsorption may also occur in bacterial overgrowth (see Chapter 9). Vitamin B_{12} is the nutrient most at risk of deficiency.

Chronic pancreatitis presents as malabsorption with undigested fat and muscle fibres in the stools. In this case added to the dietetic treatment is the total avoidance of alcohol. The diet for malabsorption may be a difficult one as it has to be constructed almost entirely from carbohydrate and protein. The diet in the appendix at the end of this chapter is suitable for the initial treatment in cases of mild to moderate severe fat malabsorption.

Surgical resection of the small intestine (e.g. as a result of thrombosis or embolism of the mesenteric vessels or severe Crohn's disease or, less commonly, perforation and peritonitis caused by chronic ulceration or penetrating abdominal wounds) can lead to malabsorption and secondary malnutrition. It is, nevertheless, possible to maintain good nutrition with remarkably little small intestine, in some cases no more than 1–2 m.

Radiation therapy and treatment with folate antagonists for cancer may worsen the cachectic effects of malignancies. Chronic regional enteritis (Crohn's disease) is another cause of diarrhoea with nutritional consequences.

Clinical aspects

An important part of the management of the nutritional consequences of diarrhoea is making the appropriate diagnosis. The underlying cause of the diarrhoea will influence the type of nutritional problems that are likely to be present and will certainly affect the management. Diet plays a larger part in the management of diarrhoea of noninfectious origin as, for example, in coeliac disease. Any significant changes in weight should be enquired into and, in general, a sudden unexplained and unintended weight loss, even though it may not be very great, may be of great importance.

Important factors in the management of the elderly patient's nutritional problem include recognition of the dependence on others for shopping, food preparation and feeding, and social factors such as having someone who can help in cases when the diarrhoea worsens. Other relevant considerations are changes in dietary patterns, new or changed dentition and other problems with eating.

The mainstay of therapy is appropriate fluid and electrolyte replacement. In nontoxic, nonbacteraemic patients, routine use of antibiotics is not indicated. Antimicrobial therapy does not substitute for aggressive supportive care, including hydration and maintenance of normal acid–base status. Fluid replacement with oral rehydration solutions containing 3.5 g sodium chloride, 2.9 g trisodium citrate dihydrate, 1.5 g potassium chloride and 20 g glucose per litre of water is well tolerated and adequate in most circumstances.

Dietary intake can be considerably decreased in diarrhoea. Less food also tends to be eaten during episodes of fever. It may therefore be necessary to advise the patient to eat small amounts more frequently and to ensure that the food is as attractively presented as possible and to encourage increased consumption of oral fluids.

Constipation with impaction and overflow can be treated by increasing the fluid and the fibre content of the diet (see Chapters 6 and 17)

Fibre is important, particularly in alleviating constipation and diverticular disease, and contributing to a more mixed diet. Nevertheless, while helpful in the management of constipation, diabetes and hyperlipidaemia, a high fibre diet can also chelate some minerals and increase faecal loss of calcium, iron, magnesium and zinc, and cause flatulence. Reduction of intraluminal colonic pressure and transit time with increasing bulk is beneficial in the treatment of irritable colon and diverticular disease.

A question that needs to be asked in the management of nutrition in diarrhoea in the elderly is whether there is always a place for supplementation with food or vitamins.

Elderly women with a small body size and a very low intake of energy (calories) may not receive enough energy for their needs. A diet that is not supplying adequate energy will also usually be one where the intake of other nutrients is at risk. A study of nursing home patients showed that levels of ascorbic acid in the white cells of the elderly were much lower than those of young adults, and were only raised to the levels of the latter by adding 80 mg of ascorbic acid daily to their diet which, in any case, already contained some ascorbic acid.

One suggestion has been for a supplement less than the standard dose of vitamin A, but a little extra of vitamins B_6 and B_{12}, folate, zinc and calcium. Nevertheless, a poor diet is not converted to a good diet by adding a vitamin supplement.

Prevention

As always, one should not neglect the aspects of prevention. The elderly display eating habits acquired at a younger age, which have been modified by diminished physical activity and by disabilities associated with aging.

Given the association of impaired immunity in the elderly with nutritional deficiencies, nutritional counselling and a supplement result in improved indicators of immune responses. The administration of zinc is associated with improved delayed cutaneous hypersensitivity.

It is now known that elderly volunteers receiving a daily supplement of vitamins and minerals for a year have higher levels of T cells and higher antibody response to the influenza vaccine, and experience significantly less frequent infection-related illness than the placebo group. It is concluded from the evidence available that 'nutritional status is an important determinant of immunocompetence in old age and that an optimum intake of micronutrients is needed for enhanced immune responses in elderly subjects'.

Large megadoses of any vitamins are not recommended. Even in younger people there are well recognized side-effects, and the effects of long-term administration are uncertain but are likely to be, if anything, exacerbated in the elderly with the slowing down of some of the excretory systems. Elderly people seem to handle vitamin A differently from the young, probably age related or related to declining renal or hepatic function, or both, and are therefore perhaps more likely to suffer toxic effects. Indeed, it has been found that very large doses of some micronutrients may impair immunity.

The diet of older people is also important and, in particular, the need to maintain fluid intake, often at levels that might seem to be more than is necessary. A mixed diet is important, especially as psychosocial factors can sometimes lead to a relatively nonnutritious, boring diet. If food is kept at low temperatures for a long period or repeatedly reheated, water-soluble vitamins in particular can be lost. In such circumstances, food safety can also become an issue.

Prevention of infections spread by food and the faecal–oral route depends on scrupulous attention to cleanliness along the whole food chain: abattoirs, food manufacturers, warehouses, retail shops, catering establishments, restaurants and domestic kitchens. Food-borne infections and faecal–oral diseases are especially prevalent in poor urban communities with poor facilities for storing foods, inadequate water supplies and waste disposal.

Another aspect of prevention that should be considered is during travel, in which an increasing number of elderly people are participating. These aspects are discussed in Chapter 9.

There exist complex interrelationships between aging, diarrhoea and nutrition. The elderly, particularly those institutionalized, are already at some increased risk of nutritional deficiencies and infections. Diarrhoea is not uncommon and can lead to clinical malnutrition. The elderly are also at relatively greater risk of death from gastrointestinal causes. Nutritional management of diarrhoea in the elderly should include the encouragement of increased consumption of oral fluids, continued feeding and eating of appropriate diets, vitamin supplementation and a strengthening of social support systems. Prevention of future episodes by manipulating the local and personal environment of the elderly person concerned will need to be assessed and implemented.

APPENDIX

A diet for fat malabsorption

The diet for malabsorption has to be constructed almost entirely from carbohydrate and protein. The diet described below is suitable for the initial treatment in cases of mild to moderate severity.

Management

Liberal use should be made of unrefined cereals, e.g. wholemeal bread and flour, or fresh fruit, vegetables and nuts. One tablespoonful of an unprocessed bran may be taken with the breakfast cereal. Refined cereals and flours, e.g. white bread, rice, pasta, cakes and pastries, should be avoided.

People vary in their response to a high-fibre diet, and in some individuals doses of fibre should be small at first and increased gradually.

Low fat, high energy diet

Indications   For patients with malabsorption and steatorrhoea

Nutrients   Fat 45–50 g, protein 120 g, energy approx 11.7 MJ (2800 kcal); adequate in all nutrients.

Food for the day   Milk, skimmed 680–1360 ml

Lean meat, poultry, fish, 200–230 g

Bread, cereal, 8–12 slices or equivalent

Vegetables, 2–3 servings

Fruit, any with no fat

Sample daily menu

Breakfast   Fruit or fruit juice

Cereal or porridge with skimmed milk

One egg

Toast or rolls with jelly, jam or marmalade

Margarine, 7 g

Coffee or tea with skimmed milk and sugar

Mid-morning   Coffee or tea with skimmed milk and sugar

Mid-day   Fruit juice or meat soup

Lean meat or fish, 90 g

Vegetables or salad

Bread, or roll or potato

Fruit or fat-free dessert made from cereal, skimmed milk and sugar

Coffee or tea with skimmed milk and sugar

Mid-afternoon   Tea with skimmed milk and sugar

Evening meal   Same as mid-day

Bedtime   Skimmed milk (flavoured) with crackers and jelly or jam

Management

The following foods should be avoided: all fried foods, organ meats, whole milk, cheese, cream and cream substitutes, ice cream, milk chocolate, cream soup, gravies, commercial cakes, pies and cookies (biscuits).

Medium-chain triglycerides can be used to increase energy intake without causing steatorrhoea. Proprietary preparations are Portagen (Mead Johnson) and MCT Oil (Cow and Gate, Liquegen). Recipes for incorporating these into food are obtainable from the manufacturers.

Boiled sweets, fruit, fruit juice and carbonated drinks may be taken.

BIBLIOGRAPHY AND FURTHER READING

Chandra, R.K. (1992). Effect of vitamin and trace-element supplementation on immune responses and infection in elderly subjects. *Lancet* **340**:1124–7.

Chandra, R.K. (1991). Nutrition and immunity in the elderly. *Nutr. Res. Rev.* **53** (4 Pt 2):580–3; discussion 583–5.

Darnton-Hill, I. (1992). Psychosocial aspects of nutrition and aging. *Nutr. Rev.* **50**:476–79.

Frongillo, E.A. Jr, Rauschenbach, B.S., Roe, D.A. & Williamson, D.F. (1992). Characteristics related to elderly persons' not eating for 1 or more days: implications for meal programs. *Am. J. Public Health* **82**:600–2.

Gangarosa, R.E., Glass, R.I., Lew, J.F. & Boring, J.R .(1992). Hospitalizations involving gastroenteritis in the United States, 1985: The special burden of the disease among the elderly. *Am. J. Epidemiol.* **135**:281–90.

Holt, P.R. (1990). Diarrhoea and malabsorption in the elderly. *Gastroenterol. Clin. North Am.* **19**:345–59.

Horwitz, A., MacFayden, D.M., Munro, H., Scrimshaw, N.S., Sten, B. & Williams, T.F. (1989). *Nutrition in the Elderly*. Oxford: Oxford University Press.

Lew, J.F., Glass, R.I., Gangarosa, R.E., Cohen, I.P., Bern, C. & Moe, C.L. (1991). Diarrhoeal deaths in the United States, 1979 through 1987. A special problem for the elderly. *J. Am. Med. Assoc.* **265**:3280–4.

Manson, A. & Shea, S. (1991). Malnutrition in elderly ambulatory medical patients. *Am. J. Public Health* **81**:1195–7.

Munro, H.N. (1981). Nutrition and ageing. *Br. Med. Bull.* **37**:83–8.

Passmore, R. & Eastwood, M.A. (1986). *Human Nutrition and Dietetics*, 8th edn ed. L.S.P. Davidson, R. Passmore & M.A. Eastwood. Edinburgh: Churchill Livingstone.

Review (1990). Practical nutritional advice for the elderly, Part I: Evaluation, supplements, RDAs. A Geriatrics Panel Discussion. *Geriatrics* **45**:26–31, 34.

Review (1990). Practical nutritional advice for the elderly, Part II: Modification and motivation. A Geriatrics Panel Discussion. *Geriatrics* **45**:47–9, 52–4, 57.

Warne, R.W. & Prinsley, D.M. (eds.) (1988). *A Manual of Geriatric Care*. Sydney: Williams & Wilkins.

The nursing care of older people with diarrhoea and constipation

Tina Koch, Pamela F. Sando and Sally Hudson

Introduction

The subjects of diarrhoea and constipation are often the source of hilarity. Anglo-Saxon culture has a rich tradition of 'lavatory' language and humour, which most people indulge in at times. It is reasonable to think, however, that one group of people who are not entertained by such humour are those people most affected by these conditions – i.e. themselves, or their carers.

Diarrhoea and constipation are often considered to be common among older people yet there is little research that addresses these and the related problems of faecal incontinence and excessive flatus. The notion that these conditions are a normal consequence of aging cannot be supported yet is widely believed in the general community.

It is unfortunate that many health care providers also hold the belief that older people are normally incontinent of faeces or, alternatively, have a 'bowel fixation' which leads to frequent complaints of constipation. These ideas reflect stereotypical attitudes about age and contribute to ageist prejudice that trivializes quite real concerns. This, in turn, can lead to individuals being reluctant to acknowledge that they have a problem, either from feelings of humiliation or fear of further ridicule. Norton (1994) says that the problems of diarrhoea and faecal incontinence are '. . . significantly under-reported symptoms which many . . . accept and disguise because of shame and embarrassment . . . [and that] . . . most people with faecal incontinence receive no professional help'.

Faecal incontinence and flatus are associated with both diarrhoea and constipation. It is often not recognized that faecal incontinence can be a result of constipation, rather than diarrhoea. This can have the result of the client being treated inappropriately, and measures to control diarrhoea being implemented, with potentially distressing outcomes.

The plan of nursing care for people with diarrhoea and/or constipation must be based on the premise that these are symptoms rather than disease entities in themselves. They are multifactorial in causation. Therefore, intervention must be directed towards eliminating the causes, rather than just dealing with the symptoms. Planning for nursing care must also include recognition of the impact of these bowel problems on the individual as a whole. Attention should be focused on the psychosocial implications of what is often seen as an embarrassing, if not shameful, problem. Shortsighted, symptomatic treatment, in the absence of rigorous assessment, will only lead to a recurring problem, with dissatisfaction for both nurse and client.

Before an assessment can be made, it is essential to have a clear understanding of what diarrhoea and constipation mean to the patient or carer. Many people believe that they are constipated if they do not have a daily bowel evacuation. While normal bowel elimination can vary from two to three times a day to two to three times a week, it is more helpful to know the individual's definition of diarrhoea and constipation. It is essential that any reported change in an older person's bowel habits should be taken seriously. All changes in normal bowel habits should be considered suspect until proven otherwise. This is particularly important in long-term residential and community nursing care. In acute care, changes in bowel habits can often be attributed to drug side-effects, dietary changes, decreased mobility, abdominal or anorectal surgery and decreased oral fluid intake. Nevertheless, if the problem does not resolve within two to three days, further investigations should be considered.

The environment in which nursing care takes place can vary from the home to the acute care setting, or nursing home or hostels. Regardless of where that may be, the primary goals of care must be to:

- assess the nature and extent of the problem
- identify the causative factors whenever possible, while recognizing that some causes may never be found
- assess their effects on the individual
- restore clients to their normal state of functioning with minimal delay consistent with good nursing practice
- institute a health education programme which has as its emphasis a discovery learning approach. This enables clients or their carers to experience for themselves the significant benefits of often quite small changes in behaviour. Many of the causes of diarrhoea can be prevented with adequate education. An education programme is a priority.

Adequate education about the effects of certain drugs on the body system needs to be provided for the older person. It must be stressed that any diarrhoea resulting from medication use should be treated promptly. The physician and the nurse are responsible for providing this education whenever new drugs are prescribed. The client should also be taught about the ill-effects of prolonged laxative use, emphasizing that control of bowel function can usually be more safely achieved through dietary control.

A focus on diet and its influence in bowel control and motility is important. The nurse needs to emphasize the importance of a healthy diet which is high in fibre content, and contains fresh fruit and vegetables. Plenty of water, fresh air and exercise will enhance the health of the individual and keep the bowel healthy and functioning normally.

Another widely held belief about older people is that they are no longer able to learn. This myth has as much validity as the myth that most, if not all, older people are incontinent, or are bowel fixated. Because many older people believe this particular piece of nonsense too, the discovery *and* experiential approach is especially useful and effective.

Diarrhoea

Diarrhoea is a distressing condition at any age, but its effects on older people can be severe and incapacitating both physically and psychologically in a comparatively short space of time. Elderly people have a reduced ability to maintain homeostasis. Elderly patients are at greater risk of dehydration and shock than a younger person is in the same circumstances. The fear of not reaching the toilet in time and the distress if faecal incontinence does occur can engender feelings of self disgust and distrust in ability to cope with daily living. Diarrhoea and faecal incontinence in older people can often lead to the abandonment of home care, leading to nursing home placement.

Dietary indiscretion is one of the most common causes of acute diarrhoea. This can be anything from too much fruit or highly spiced or rich food, contaminated food due to improper storage, or even unaccustomed overindulgence in alcohol. Other prominent aetiological factors are discussed elsewhere in this text. Acute-onset diarrhoea as a result of bacterial contamination due to *Staphylococcus, E. coli* or viral infection – Norwalk and Rotavirus for example – can be life threatening. For this reason, acute-onset diarrhoea within an institution needs immediate investigation and treatment. Older people living at home also need to be aware of the danger of diarrhoea which does not resolve, and seek medical assistance.

Chronic diarrhoea can be insidious in onset. It can often be interspersed with periods of normal bowel movement or constipation, and therefore not seen as a problem. Again, the elderly person may attribute the diarrhoea to a dietary cause ('something I ate'). Frequent faecal staining which cannot be attributed to inadequate cleaning may be the first sign that something more serious than the occasional episode of self-limiting diarrhoea has developed. Embarrassment and sensitivity about bowel control will often prevent people seeking help and treatment until more severe consequences occur.

The causes of chronic diarrhoea range from infectious causes (see Chapters 8 and 9) to malabsorption due to coeliac disease (see Chapter 11). A major cause of diarrhoea among elderly people is adverse reactions to drugs due to increased consumption of drugs. Laxative overuse must always be considered as a cause of chronic diarrhoea.

Constipation

Constipation and diarrhoea have been labelled 'the neglected symptoms'. There is evidence that millions of dollars are spent annually on over-the-counter medications to seek relief from constipation. A common perception among many health care providers is that older people are constipated as a direct result of aging. One of the major causes of this perception is the increased use of laxative preparations by older people, often as a self-prescribed item. There is good evidence that there is no relationship between aging and changes in bowel motility. Laxatives continue to be unnecessarily prescribed even though some laxatives can have damaging effects if used habitually. It has been suggested that a cascade of contributing factors can be implicated in older people's use of laxatives. Another major factor is thought to be advertising directed at older people.

The key to identifying causes of constipation lies in thorough assessment of clients and their lifestyle. Older clients are often distressed by constipation, and may complain of headaches, malaise, abdominal discomfort and bloating. The causes of constipation, as with diarrhoea, are many (see Chapter 16). They can range from drug side-effects and intrinsic gastrointestinal tract disorders, to lack of privacy, habitual ignoring of the call to stool and habitual laxative use. A common cause is self-imposed inadequate fluid intake, in the mistaken belief that this is an effective way to manage urgency or urinary incontinence.

The nurse's role

Nurses have an important role in the care of an older person with diarrhoea and constipation. Faecal excretion is a very private function. Control is usually established in about the second year of life and then maintained. An important aspect of care is to support the client's right to keep as much control as possible over their situation. This requires an attempt to manage the problems at home, with help from family members and/or a domiciliary nursing care service. The benefits of this approach include avoidance of the stress and regimentation that a hospital admission imposes and, more importantly, avoidance of the nosocomial infections common following hospital admission.

For many years nurses have, either formally or informally, used what has come to be known as the 'nursing process' as a framework for developing and implementing plans of care. The client's involvement in this cyclical process of assessment, nursing diagnosis, planning, intervention and evaluation is crucial for optimum client outcome.

Assessment

Sound client assessment is fundamental to the process of planning and delivery of nursing care. This requires an interview and a physical assessment to establish a baseline and to develop a plan of care. Assessment requires an ability to build rapport and gain the client's trust, in addition to skilful use of observation and data gathering techniques. Assessment is a continuous process, which is only completed when no further nursing care is needed.

The extent of alterations in a person's lifestyle is an important part of the nursing assessment. Diarrhoea is a particular threat to independent older people. They may feel weak and less able to carry out the activities of daily living. If bowel control is difficult they will be afraid to move too far from a toilet, and are unlikely to welcome visitors. This can result in social isolation. There is also the potential for malnutrition due to reduced food intake in the mistaken belief that 'resting the gut' will control the problem.

Sufficient time must be set aside for the initial interview and assessment. Sensory loss, such as visual and/or hearing impairment, will prolong the interview and make it more difficult for both the nurse and the client. An approach to taking a history from an older person is discussed in Chapter 4. A private area which includes facilities to perform a physical examination, and which allows discussion to take place without being overheard, is essential.

Whichever interview tool is used, it must be versatile enough to enable the collection of general information such as:

- personal data
- past and present health history; for women, this should include obstetrical history
- relevant family history and drug consumption of both prescribed and over-the-counter medications.

The more specific history should include

- onset and duration of symptoms
- presence, location and character of any pain
- food and fluid intake
- frequency and character of faecal output
- associated problems, e.g. painful excoriation, especially around the perianal area due to frequent contact with faecal matter.

If, for example due to dementia, the client is unable to communicate adequately, information should be obtained from the carer. This adds another dimension to the assessment and management of a client with a bowel dysfunction living at home.

The carer is commonly of a comparable age to the client and may not have the strength to undertake the physically demanding tasks associated with managing bowel care. The carer may have to enlist assistance.

The carer working alone or with assistance needs support from the nurse, who is also able to refer to other community agencies for assistance. Depending on the wishes of the carer and, if possible the client, respite care can also be arranged.

Physical assessment

The physical assessment process must be discussed with the client, and agreement obtained. The assessment of dehydration is discussed in Chapter 4 and, due to the distinct differences between the signs in young patients and the elderly, bears repetition here.

The immediate concern in the elderly patient is to decide if dehydration or hypovolaemia is present. The conventional criteria are reduction of skin turgor, increased thirst, decreased peripheral perfusion, postural hypotension, low jugular vein pressure, patient sensation of thirst and dryness, tachycardia and temperature. There is now evidence that these signs may be unreliable in the elderly. Gross et. al. (1992) conducted a prospective, correlational study with 55 subjects aged 60 or older, and concluded that these conventional signs and symptoms (derived from younger patients) of dehydration are unreliable in the elderly patient. None of these symptoms or signs were strong correlates of dehydration in the elderly. The reasons for the lack of correlation are that there are normal age-related changes in these variables, and that the physiological responses to dehydration vary markedly between the elderly and younger patients. For example, postural hypotension is a common sign in the elderly patient, independent of the state of hydration, due to autonomic dysfunction and drug therapy.

Seven signs and symptoms are highlighted that strongly correlate with dehydration in the elderly, but are independent of significant, age-related change. They are:
- dry tongue
- longitudinal tongue furrows
- dry mucous membranes of nose and mouth
- eyes that appear recessed in their sockets
- upper body muscle weakness
- speech difficulty
- confusion.

Although the nutritional status and dietary intake will have been discussed during the initial interview, the physical assessment provides the opportunity for the nurse to consider the general physical condition of the patient, and assess the urgency of any intervention.

Auscultation of the abdomen for bowel sounds (with a *warm* stethoscope) is performed before palpation or percussion. Warm hands are also necessary for abdominal percussion and palpation, to prevent tensing of the abdominal muscles, which makes palpation difficult and causes unnecessary pain. Following percussion, the client's hands are placed on the abdomen and covered with the nurse's. Palpation is begun gently while the muscles relax. Once relaxed, the client's hands are removed. It is important to ask which areas are painful. These areas are palpated last.

The rectal examination is of particular importance in the assessment of anorectal problems. While it is usually considered undignified (at best) by clients, it can provide a great deal of information. A full explanation of the need and process must be given, and consent obtained. Before the rectal examination the anal area is checked for anal fissures, haemorrhoids and rectal prolapse. The perianal area is inspected for signs of 'nappy rash' or thickened skin, which could indicate a long-standing problem. After this inspection the rectum can be checked with a well lubricated, gloved finger. Rectal contents, sphincter strength and pelvic muscle strength can all be assessed with this procedure.

Other data-gathering tools include bowel, fluid balance and weight charts. Continuing weight loss can indicate dehydration or inadequate food intake. A record of bowel actions, including times and character, should be maintained whether the client is in hospital, supported care or at home. It can be kept by the client, carer or nurse. This information can often be correlated with other factors such as food or fluid intake. Testing for occult blood is essential, especially for patients with chronic diarrhoea.

When data has been collected, the nursing diagnoses are made. Decisions regarding treatment are taken in collaboration with the client's medical practitioner. The nursing care plan is developed in collaboration with the client and carer. The plan of care will incorporate the client's normal elimination behaviours, habits and routines.

Planning nursing care

Nursing care for the older person with diarrhoea is determined by several factors:

- the severity of the diarrhoea
- the effects on the client and the client's carer
- the influence other disease processes may have – or vice versa
- the severity of dehydration, electrolyte imbalance and nutritional deficit.

The goal of nursing care at home must be to maintain independence and control of bowel actions in familiar surroundings. The client or carer monitoring the problem, with the assistance of the district nurse as needed, may avoid admission to hospital. Hospital admission is ideally considered only as a last resort.

Nutrition is a major consideration when planning care. Some deviation from normal diet may initially be necessary to control the diarrhoea. If a dietary item such as gluten is implicated, as in coeliac disease (see Chapter 11), permanent dietary changes are necessary. After rehydration and stabilization, dietary modification in the form of increased fibre is indicated to maintain optimal bowel function.

Poor nutritional status will have an impact on any pre-existing health problems and also increase the health risks associated with diarrhoea. There is an increased risk of skin breakdown from the effects of the stool on the perianal area, and for the development of pressure sores in clients who are debilitated or confined to bed.

Implementation of nursing care

The nursing care to be implemented will depend on the cause of the diarrhoea, and its actual and potential effect on the elderly person. Intervention strategies are based on body weight, skin condition and laboratory findings used to assess nutrition, hydration and electrolyte status.

Depending on aetiology, the implementation of nursing care may involve:

- treating the diarrhoea with therapeutic agents
- dietary modifications
- rehydration
- bowel training, if possible, if the problem is a chronic one
- enemas if necessary
- manual removal (if impaction is the cause).

Aspects of nursing care which are adjuncts to medical therapy, include testing of the stool for occult blood, collection of faecal specimens for the laboratory, and patient preparation for any investigations. These tests could include barium enema or colonoscopy (both of which require specific bowel preparation), upper gastrointestinal endoscopy and small intestinal biopsy.

Rehydration can often be achieved with an adequate and appropriate oral fluid intake. Intravenous therapy will only be needed if dehydration and electrolyte imbalance cannot be managed more conservatively. In the more severe cases of diarrhoea it is important to monitor the fluid status, electrolyte levels and serum albumin. There may be reluctance on the part of the patient to eat and drink, believing that this will aggravate the diarrhoea. The need to reassure clients that food and fluids will cause no harm cannot be overemphasized.

In the hospital setting as much consideration as possible must be given to assist the client to maintain independence and control over bowel function. This is difficult to achieve in an institutional environment. Routines and shared facilities imposed by institutions often require a sacrifice of privacy, dignity and independence. Communal toilet facilities which are situated some distance from beds are not conducive to controlling incontinence or reducing anxiety. These problems are compounded in patients with dementia. Efforts should be made to ensure that the older person with diarrhoea is as close as possible to the toilet.

If the client is cognitively impaired, important strategies for nursing management are scheduled for toileting, especially after meals to take advantage of the gastrocolic reflex, ensuring adequate privacy and that devices to protect against soiling of clothes (such as disposable briefs and incontinence pads) are implemented.

A comprehensive programme of bowel training is necessary for those who have lost sphincter control and have a significant incontinence problem. The aim of the training programme should be to promote defaecation at approximately the same time each day, consistent with normal elimination. Sensory retraining programmes have been advocated for those clients who have faecal incontinence and meet the assessment criteria for a probable successful outcome. Criteria for success include ability to ambulate, intact cognitive functioning and the discipline to carry out the programme requirements. While many existing treatment programmes are helpful, sensory retraining offers a cost-effective programme which can be managed by advanced practice nurses in the community. Positive encouragement of the client's progress should be part of the nursing involvement as it may take several weeks for the programme to be successful.

Containment

A useful adjunct in the management of faecal incontinence is the recently developed 'anal plug'. The product has potential for people who are reluctant to wear a nappy. The plug can be worn for up to twelve hours. At first sight it looks like a short tampon, but within seconds of insertion it moulds to a mushroom shape within the rectum. Lying just above the internal anal sphincter, it blocks egress of faecal matter until it is removed. The plug is covered with a soft, knitted fabric extending into a 'tail' about 10 cm in length that hangs outside the body. This enables easy removal when necessary. The benefits of such a product are obvious for a client who is not bedbound, or otherwise incapable of benefiting from such a product. Sadly, some clinical nurse advisers have reported that several of their elderly clients have been unable to even consider using such a device, even though their quality of life has been profoundly affected by faecal incontinence.

Collection pads are available from various outlets. Some manufacturers have also developed schemes where clients are able to order by telephone, and receive supplies delivered to the door, for a small fee in addition to the normal cost. People considering using these devices should ideally be referred to a continence nurse adviser for in-depth assessment and management advice. These pads have a number of disadvantages, including: the need for removal as soon as they become soiled, to prevent skin damage; the cost of the product; adequate disposal strategies; and odour, which can be embarrassing for the client.

Another option is the faecal collection bag. These are only useful for bedbound clients. Hair around the perianal area must be removed, and the bag is applied. In appearance it is similar to a colostomy bag, and performs the same function. Some people find them difficult to apply and keep in place.

Skin care

Skin care, including regular skin assessment, is another important part of nursing care. The focus is on protecting the perineal area from exposure to faeces and checking skin integrity. In the independent older person, it is necessary to ensure access to warm water, mild soaps and emollient creams so that adequate, gentle, skin cleansing can be carried out after each bowel action. The nurse will be responsible for that care in the dependent person. The perineal area should be inspected to detect a break in the integrity of the skin surface, and secondary infections such as candida, which can occur in the already compromised patient. Skin protection barriers (e.g. Stomahesive type powder or wipes) can often be of benefit.

Tube feeding

Tube feeding of older people is often limited to the hospital setting but with increasing support systems clients needing this type of feeding are more frequently being cared for at home. Acute diarrhoea as a result of tube feeding can be related to the volume and rate of administration of the formula, its osmolarity and composition.

Diarrhoea can be caused by the volume of the formula being administered and usually occurs when the formula regime commences. If the feeds are commenced at a low volume and increased gradually diarrhoea is unlikely to occur. Diarrhoea is less of a problem since the introduction of formulas containing fibre. Initial high volumes can, however, cause a type of 'dumping syndrome' in some clients, where the gut is unable to absorb the large protein and nutrient load. If this does occur, the feed is excreted from the bowel with minimal absorption of the nutritional elements. This phenomenon tends to be more marked in the person with poor underlying nutritional status.

It has been thought that the temperature of the formula influences the absorption, and formulas that are administered cold from the refrigerator will induce diarrhoea. It is therefore advisable to have the formula at room temperature before administration. Heating the formula is not recommended as it has been shown to increase the risk of bacterial contamination of feeds and can subsequently cause diarrhoea.

Faecal impaction

There is no evidence to suggest that constipation or impaction is inevitable with aging, but certain risk factors occur more frequently in the older population. The risks are associated with prolonged inactivity, immobility or decreased mobility, inability to communicate the need for defaecation to health care workers or carers, environmental factors including deviation from the usual routine, and side-effects of medication usage.

Impaction may occur in the hospital or residential care setting for a number of reasons. Immobilization (sometimes unnecessarily), a change of environment, loss of privacy and an inability to sit up in bed on a bedpan to defaecate are all common, and usually preventable, factors which can be implicated. Dietary changes, underlying medical conditions, anxiety and alterations to normal patterns of bowel control constitute further reasons.

Faecal impaction is usually the result of chronic constipation, and may present as a mucous, diarrhoea-like discharge which seeps around the faecal mass (see Chapter 6). This may be observed as faecal incontinence in the elderly client. If faecal impaction is suspected, a rectal examination will confirm this, as hard faeces can be felt digitally in the rectum in 98 per cent of cases. Treatment involves a course of enemas until the colon is cleared. This may be checked by plain abdominal radiography. If these measures fail, manual disimpaction will become necessary.

The patient's comfort and privacy must be ensured during the process of disimpaction. A complete explanation about the procedure must be given and consent obtained. Analgesia may be required in addition to a local anaesthetic to the anorectal tissue before the removal of faeces. A warm mineral oil enema given before the procedure may serve to make the faeces easier to remove. The impacted faeces may have to be removed in stages depending on the person's level of tolerance. Adequate time should be allowed for rest, in between removal of portions of stool, reassurance given and close observation made for any untoward effects. The process may need to be repeated on subsequent days with the administration of concurrent mild laxatives and daily or twice daily enemas. The entire procedure and its result is recorded in the nursing notes.

The most common nursing treatment option for diarrhoea secondary to constipation or impaction is the administration of an enema. Enemas are a successful treatment option. The choice of enema lies mainly with the individual preference of the nurse or medical officer. Choices are usually made between microlax (or similar) and glycerine and oil (G & O) enemas. These are aimed at lubricating the area around the impacted faeces, allowing for easier passage from the rectum. G & O enemas consist of equal parts of glycerine and olive oil; and water warm enough to bring the enema to blood temperature (36 °C) before administration. Usually there is 90 to 100 ml of each constituent, although this can be modified if necessary following assessment.

Microlax is one of the commercially available microenemas. These are more useful for minor defaecation problems than impaction. They are faecal softeners which liberate water from the stool, causing a softening of the outside of the stool to facilitate gentle defaecation. There is no place for the old fashioned soap and water enema. Its use has been shown to damage the bowel mucosa, and recommendations for administration are to be deplored.

Before an enema is administered, the client must be informed about the procedure and encouraged to retain the enema for as long as possible. This will allow maximum softening of the stool to take place. It is also important that there is ready and easy access to a toilet or commode to prevent loss of control, and embarrassment to the individual. The process of enema administration will stimulate peristaltic movement and sphincter relaxation to empty the bowel.

Nursing care of the client with constipation

The care of a client complaining of constipation is similar to that of caring for a client with diarrhoea. Dietary modification, increasing the fibre and fluid content of the diet and education are the mainstays of care. Several factors are considered to be implicated in the development of constipation. While not all of these factors can be modified, for example immobility of a frail, aged client, there is evidence that for most clients, laxatives must be considered a last resort. Constipation can be effectively managed based on a philosophy of health education, regular exercise within the capabilities of the individual and timely toileting for those at risk.

Evaluation

The effectiveness of the nursing care is measured by the degree of success in achieving the expected outcomes. This would ideally occur with the return of the older person to normal bowel function, and also provide adequate information about the risks associated with alteration in bowel function. The elderly person's return to an independent life is of course the ultimate desired outcome.

Nursing care of the older person with diarrhoea or constipation is a significant nursing challenge and must be aimed primarily at identifying the cause, reducing the associated risks and maintaining independence and control. The aim is to restore normal bowel function and to maintain a high quality of life of the elderly person. This requires a collaborative approach between the older person, the physician and the nurse.

APPENDIX I

Food Contamination

Nearly 50 per cent of all episodes of diarrhoea are associated with food-borne illnesses caused by improper food handling. The risks associated with diarrhoea from infections and contaminated foods can be minimized by education about the modes of transmission of organisms and sound food preparation and storage practices.

The nurse will need to instigate an educational and preventative programme to reduce the recurrence of episodes of diarrhoea secondary to food contamination. Community health nurses and district nurses are in an excellent position to implement such a programme. The main points to emphasize include:

- handwashing before handling food
- thawing food in the refrigerator
- washing hands, utensils and surfaces after contact with raw meat or poultry
- leaving perishable food out of the refrigerator for a maximum of two hours
- refrigerating or freezing leftovers promptly.

The risks associated with diarrhoea from infections and contaminated foods can be minimized by education about the modes of transmission of organisms and sound food preparation practices.

APPENDIX II

Defaecation assessment: questions to the older person

Bowel actions

What term do you use to describe defaecation? e.g. bowel action or bowel function or going to the lavatory or going to the loo or dunny

(Use the term preferred by the person for the following questions).

- What concerns you most about this symptom? e.g. incontinence, offended by smell, embarrassment about the mess, embarrassment at communicating need to defaecate, inability to reach the lavatory, difficulty in removing clothes, difficulty in wiping the bottom because of arthritic hands, feeling weak
- What is the usual pattern of defaecation?
- What do you understand by the term constipation?
- How often do you have your bowels open?

- Do you have constipation?
- What happens when you need to defaecate? e.g. do you have a sensation
- Do you experience urgency?
- Do you have any time of warning?
- How long do you usually take to defaecate?
- Do you strain when you defaecate?
- Is defaecation associated with:
  1. Pain
  2. Bleeding (fresh or altered blood)
  3. Mucous
  4. Flatus (or preferred word)
- Can you describe the stools? e.g. Ribbon stools
- What colour are they?
- What is the consistency?
- Is the consistency different today?
- What is the usual amount of faeces?
- Is this different today? What is the amount today?
- Do you feel the rectum has been cleared?
- Has there been a change in your bowel habits recently?

Diet

- Do you take any food for your bowels?
- Do you avoid any foods?
- How much fibre do you have in a day – high or low
- How much fluid do you usually drink in one day?
- How much are you drinking today?
- Do you restrict your fluids?

Laxative use

- Do you use a laxative or opening medicine?
- What is your history of laxative use?
- Did you take any constipating medicine?
- Do you have haemorrhoids or any other problems around your anus?

Continence

- Can you hold the bowel contents until you can reach the lavatory or commode?
- Is this a problem today?

- If it is a problem, can you tell me what happens when you need to go the lavatory?
- Is there a sensation of incontinence?
- How often does this (incontinence) happen in one day (take today as an example)?
- Are you troubled by urinary incontinence?

Environment or mobility

Can you tell me about any problems with using the lavatory? e.g. walking, distance to the lavatory, ability to cleanse using the lavatory paper, flushing the lavatory?

Drugs

- Are you taking antibiotics?
- Are you taking any other medicines?
- Can I see your medicines?
- Did your doctor prescribe these?

Other history

- Can you describe your exercise routine?
- Can you tell me if you have had previous surgery of the gastrointestinal tract?
- Do you have a colostomy or ileostomy?

REFERENCES AND FURTHER READING

Abyad, A. & Mourad, F. (1996). Constipation: common sense care of the older patient. *Geriatrics* 51:28–34, 36.

Annells, M.P. (1997). *The Impact of Flatus Upon the Nurse.* Ph.D. Dissertation, Flinders University of South Australia, Adelaide.

Bentsen, D. & Braun, J.W. (1996). Controlling fecal incontinence with sensory retraining managed by advanced practice nurses. *Clin. Nurse Spec.* 10:171–5.

Gibson, C.J., Opalka, P.C., Moore, C.A., Brady, R.S. & Mion, L.C. (1995). Effectiveness of bran supplement on the bowel management of elderly rehabilitation patients. *J. Gerontol. Nurs.* 21:21–30.

Gray, M. & Burns, S.M. (1996). Continence management. *Crit. Care Nurs. Clin. North Am* 8:29–38.

Harari, D., Gurwitz, J.H., Avorn, J., Bohn, R. & Minaker, K.L. (1996). Bowel habits in relation to age and gender. Findings from the National Health Interview Survey and Clinical Implications. *Arch. Intern. Med.* 156:315–20.

Lawler, J. (1991). *Behind the Screens. Nursing, Somology, and the Problem of the Body*, 1st edn, Vol 1. Melbourne: Churchill Livingstone.

Nazarko, L. (1996). Preventing constipation in older people. *Prof. Nurse* 11:816–18.

Neal, L.J. (1995). 'Power pudding': natural laxative therapy for the elderly who are homebound. *Home Health Nurse* 13:66–71.

Norton, C. (1994). Asking simple questions: promoting continence. *Nurs. Stand* 8:3–8; quiz 10–3.

Polit, D.F. & Hungler, B.P. (1991). *Nursing Research: Principles and Methods*, 4th edn. Philadelphia: Lippincott.

Ratnaike, R.N. (1990). Diarrhoea in the elderly: epidemiological and etiological factors. *J. Gastroenterol Hepatol* 5:449–58.

Ratnaike, R.N. & Jones, T.E. (1992). Prescribing for the elderly II: Drug associated diarrhoea. *Curr. Ther.* 33:43–6

Read, N.W., Celik, A.F. & Katsinelos, P. (1995). Constipation and incontinence in the elderly. *J. Clin. Gastroenterol* 20:61–70.

Rodrigues-Fisher, L., Carlow, C., Bourguignon, C., & Good, B.V. (1993). Dietary fiber nursing intervention: prevention of constipation in older adults. *Clin. Nurs. Res.* 2:464–77.

Ross, D.G. (1993). Subjective data related to altered bowel elimination patterns among hospitalised elder and middle aged persons. *Orthop. Nurs.* 12:25–32.

Stoehr, G.P., Ganguli, M., Seaberg, E.C., Echement, D.A. & Belle, S. (1997). Over-the-counter medication use in an older rural community: the MoVIES project. *J. Am. Geriatr. Soc.* 45:158–65.

Williams, K. & Roe B. (1995). Developments in continence care. *Elder Care* 7:19–20, 22.

Wolf, Z.R. (1996). Bowel management and nursing's hidden work. *Nurs. Times* 92:26–8.

Wright, P.S. & Thomas, S.L. (1995). Constipation and diarrhea: the neglected symptoms. *Semin. Oncol. Nurs.* 11:289–97.

Index